6.

Food for the Community

Food for the
Community

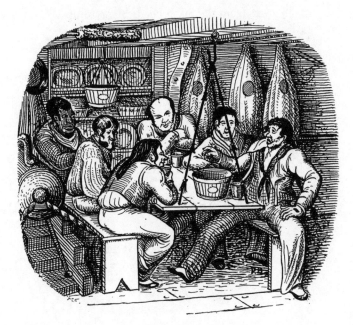

Special Diets
for
Special Groups

EDITED BY C. ANNE WILSON

Edinburgh University Press

Papers from the Sixth Leeds Symposium
on Food History and Traditions,
April 1991, with additional paper.

© C. Anne Wilson, 1993

Edinburgh University Press Ltd
22 George Square, Edinburgh

Typeset in Alphacomp Garamond
by Pioneer Associates Limited, Perthshire, and
printed in Great Britain by
The Alden Press Ltd, Oxford

A CIP record for this book is available
from the British Library

ISBN 0 7486 0431 6

Contents

Contents

About the Contributors

PETER BREARS is the Director of Leeds City Museum. He combines his interests in archaeology, architecture and the traditional food of Northern England with a great deal of practical experience of recreating the culinary confections of earlier centuries. His publications include *The Gentlewoman's Kitchen: Great Food in Yorkshire 1650-1750* and *Traditional Food in Yorkshire*.

LYNETTE MUIR, formerly a member of the French Department of the University of Leeds, is currently writing a book on *The Biblical Drama of Medieval Europe*. Her work on the domestic arrangements of the school at St Cyr developed from research for a historical school story, *The Girls of St Cyr*.

H. G. MULLER was born in Germany and came to England in 1946. He spent the first twenty years of his working life in the food industry, and is now a Senior Lecturer in the Procter Department of Food Science at the University of Leeds, where he has been teaching students since 1964. His publications include *Nutrition and Food Processing* (with G. Tobin), *Baking and Bakeries*, and *An Introduction to Tropical Food Science*.

JENNIFER STEAD was formerly lecturer in Art History at Bradford Regional College of Art. Her interests include local history – she was co-founder and is co-editor of the journal *Old West Riding* – as well as food history. Among her publications is *Food and Cooking in 18th Century Britain*.

About the Contributors

EILEEN WHITE has written about the York Mystery play and Elizabethan York. She is a local historian interested in domestic matters from the Middle Ages to the seventeenth century. She cooks regularly from old recipes, devising menus for social occasions around a period theme.

ANNE WILSON has worked for many years in the Brotherton Library of the University of Leeds, becoming involved in food history as a result of cataloguing the John Preston Collection of early English cookery books. Her publications include *Food and Drink in Britain from the Stone Age to Recent Times* and *The Book of Marmalade*. She is currently researching the very early history of distilling.

List of Illustrations

1.
Introduction

C. ANNE WILSON

Which community? That is the first question our readers will want to ask on seeing the title of this book, *Food for the Community*. The answer is that the following chapters, based on the papers given at the Sixth Leeds Symposium on Food History held in April 1991, describe the eating patterns of several different communities. When a group of people spend their time together because they are pursuing a common aim, they very often share other aspects of their daily life, among them communal meals or at least communal food provision. In such cases the provisioning arrangements have to be centralised to some degree, and records are kept to provide a yardstick for the cook, for the caterer, and for those who hold the purse strings. Foodstuffs and menus must, therefore, be standardised and repeated. The records themselves are conserved, sometimes through many years of communal eating; and several have survived for centuries.

Much source material on the history of meals takes the form of menus for special occasions – the great feasts of the medieval nobility, or the food served at festivities to celebrate a coming-of-age or wedding at a country house of the landed gentry. But the records of community meals offer a different viewpoint of food provision because they concentrate mainly on everyday catering. They give an indication of the economic status of those participating, and they also reflect rudimentary dietary theories held at the time when the community was active.

Our contributors' research brought to light some surprising dietary features. The first chapter, on monastic diet, reveals that the arrangement of the hours of the day in a medieval monastery – each hour varying in length through the year since the same number of hours had to be fitted into the period between sunrise and sunset – had a radical effect on the eating patterns of the monks. In mid-winter they received no evening meal for they went to bed at 4.30 p.m. (providing a good illustration of the old French proverb, *qui dort, dine*).

The next chapter covers the meals of servants. Some readers may wonder why this body of workers should be regarded as a community at all since they were attached to individual families, and it might be expected that they could make do on the leftovers from the families' meals. But in past centuries the servants in great households were numbered not just in tens but in scores and sometimes in hundreds, and elaborate arrangements were made to issue them with meals to reflect their rank within their own pecking order. Delicious leftovers did reach some of them, but only those holding particular designated offices.

A chapter on naval food from 1530 to 1830 follows – containing the most horrendous diets in this book. Yet the sailors clung to their salt beef, consuming it in large quantities (the quantity of meat issued to sailors drew hungry labourers to forsake the land and take to the sea), and showing little desire to copy the diet of Dutch and French sailors, who ate far less meat and fish but more cheese and butter, much less that of Spanish and Italian sailors whose basic foods were rice, oatmeal, olives, olive oil, and figs.

The boarding-school diet is represented in the following chapter by an account of the arrangements at a very unusual school, probably the oldest girls' boarding-school in Europe. It was established at St Cyr, near Versailles, through the good offices of Madame de Maintenon, morganatic wife of King Louis XIV of France, for the daughters of the impoverished nobility. There has been no equivalent to this school in Britain, for in the past the British aristocracy has been well supported by its broad acres of land, and any members who lost their wealth were left to get along as best they could. In France, however, the importance of high rank was maintained through the generations, even where the family experienced extreme poverty; and it was to support and educate the daughters of such families that the school at St Cyr was founded and funded. Some boarding-schools of later times earned a reputation for parsimony in food matters. But at St Cyr girls with good appetites were encouraged to eat heartily and enjoy their meals.

In Britain paupers who were totally unable to support themselves were catered for within institutions over a period of nearly 350 years. The next chapter discusses the provisioning of the poor-houses, which, under their later name of workhouses, continued until after the Second World War. It may come as a surprise to many readers that in their earlier manifestation as poor-houses they provided their inmates with substantial meals which contrasted favourably with the food available to many ordinary people who, through the poor rate, were forced to contribute to the inmates' upkeep.

The final chapter is an addition to the papers given at the 1991 Leeds Symposium on Food History, and its theme is army catering from the Napoleonic Wars to the Gulf War of 1991. The history of the provisioning of armies reflects the history of food preservation during the period, since preserved foods supplied a significant part of the military diet when soldiers campaigned far from their home base. The chapter also shows how the army diet was gradually modified in the light of discoveries about vitamins made during the earlier twentieth century.

Food for the Community examines areas of food history hitherto overlooked, or at least noted rather briefly in passing. The detailed accounts of the feeding of large groups of people in earlier centuries give interesting glimpses into the everyday life of those people, and show how, in many cases, members of a community were better nourished than some of their contemporaries responsible for feeding themselves in the world outside. If life within the community tended to curtail personal freedom, at least it sometimes improved the physical wellbeing of its members.

C. Anne Wilson
November 1992

2.

The Measure of the Meat: Monastic Diet in Medieval England

EILEEN WHITE

The monastic way of life can be traced back to a time before the earliest Rules identified it in the fifth and sixth centuries. In England it ended with the Dissolution of the Monasteries in the mid-sixteenth century. Over a thousand years society developed and changed, and so did the various orders of monks and nuns. The 'medieval monastic diet', even when confined to England, is thus a large subject: monasteries were founded in all parts of the country, and information about them comes piecemeal from a long period of time. Too many examples plucked from different places and times can become confusing, and generalisations can be misleading. Examples for this study are therefore taken from only a few monasteries and priories, and illustrate not so much England as Yorkshire.

Bolton Priory is situated on the banks of the River Wharfe above Ilkley. This house of the Augustinians, or Black Canons, was originally founded at Embsay, near Skipton, in 1120, and in 1155 transferred to its present site. The accounts of the Priory between 1286 and 1325 have been analysed by Ian Kershaw,[1] and are used here. The Augustinian Order developed from the Colleges of clergy serving cathedrals or collegiate churches, who lived in a community under a common discipline. A regime was laid down from the eighth century, but by the twelfth century, in reply to the Benedictines, the clerics had adopted a Rule based on that set out by St Augustine in a letter to a nunnery, about 423 AD. The Augustinians aimed at moderation, and were less strict than the Benedictines.[2]

Esholt Priory was a small Cistercian Nunnery dating from the twelfth century, situated north of Bradford on the bend of the River Aire between Bradford and Leeds. Nothing of the buildings remains now apart from remnants incorporated into the present Esholt Hall; but inventories and accounts from 1360 to 1365 have been published, and there is a detailed description of the building at the time of the Dissolution.[3]

Marrick Priory was another Nunnery, founded by the Benedictines in 1156-8 near Richmond, North Yorkshire. Its accounts for the year 1415-16 have been transcribed by John H. Tillotson.[4]

Selby Abbey is on the River Ouse, south of its junction with the Wharfe. It was founded about 1070 by the Benedictines, or Black Monks, and only the church now remains. There is, however, a good sample of account rolls remaining, and a selection of the best has been translated and published, also by Tillotson.[5] The rolls were kept by a succession of monks put in charge of various offices for a year; the main ones noted here are:

1398-9	Bursars' account (two monks) – the bursars had overall supervision of monastic expenditure, and the Abbot's expenses
1404-05	Granger's account – the granger was responsible for grain, and the associated bread and ale
1413-14	Extern Cellarer's account – the extern cellarer purchased livestock
1416-17	Kitchener's account – the kitchener was in charge of kitchen supplies; he received the provisions and kept a note of what was used. Tillotson says of this particular account that 'it remains the most impressive

single piece of evidence for the provisioning and dietary lifestyle of Selby Abbey that has survived'.[6]

Kirkstall Abbey was one of the Yorkshire houses of the Cistercians, or White Monks. This order broke away from the contemporary Benedictines to return to the more austere ideals of the Rule of St Benedict, founding its first abbey at Citeaux in 1098. Building abbeys in remote places, the monks employed lay brothers to develop and farm the outlying granges. Kirkstall was a daughter house of Fountains Abbey, and the monks first attempted to settle at Barnoldswick in 1147. In 1152 they moved down the Aire Valley to a more amenable site, already called Kirkstall, and their former house became a grange. Less renowned than its sister houses in Yorkshire, because it now stands in the suburbs of Leeds, Kirkstall is nevertheless a fascinating architectural site, retaining buildings from the initial building period, which was completed by 1182.[7] No example is noted here of the Carthusians, the most austere of the monastic Orders, with no need for later reformation.[8]

The dates of these examples should be kept in mind; there had been 500 years of life under the Benedictine Rule before the above Monasteries were established in England, and the chosen accounts themselves come from a time 160 to 370 years after the foundation of the particular community. The examples also represent a period of more than 130 years, after which monasticism in England had just over 100 years of existence left.

Monasteries were self-contained communities, enclosed to be free of distractions. They can, however, be compared with other large households of the same period which were divided into offices or departments, each needing organisation and accounts. The monks were expected to do some manual work, but their main duty was to perform regular services

The Monastic Community

in the monastic church, and over the years they became increasingly literate and scholarly, with less time for other tasks. They received gifts of money and land, and so became wealthy. The Cistercians tried to return to the original ideals of monasticism, including physical work, and they accepted gifts of land in isolated places, often considered waste, which they cultivated and made productive. However, even they needed help; and their Monasteries originally included a large proportion of lay brothers, usually illiterate men, who worked at the distant granges and who were not expected to attend the daily services in the monastic church.

The hard work of the Cistercians, along with a coherent management ultimately derived from the annual General Chapter at Cîteaux, brought them success: 'They embraced poverty but their industry made them rich. They worked so well that they soon had a surplus of food, wool, leather and other commodities. They began to come back into the world, to trade, to own money and to become worldly.'[9] It is not surprising that the largest surviving medieval barn in the country, at Great Coxwell in Oxfordshire, was built by the Cistercians.[10]

Images of plenty should not be over-emphasised, however, for the monks were not enclosed from natural or other disasters. Bolton Priory experienced failures of harvest in 1315 and 1316 after torrential rain, and their sheep flock was decimated. This was followed in 1319 and 1320 by a cattle murrain; and invasions by the Scots devastated land around Skipton. In 1320 there was a temporary dispersal of the canons, although it seems that one had to return because his host priory found it difficult to provide for even one extra mouth. The community was back in residence by 1325.[11]

Property and Exploitation

Initially, the monks exploited their property directly, with the aid of the lay brothers; from the later fourteenth century they tended to rent out the more distant land, retaining only a home farm for domestic produce.[12] They also received income from houses and other buildings bequeathed to them. All this gave them non-monastic responsibilities, and their accounts included expenses for repairs, hedging and ditching, and the maintenance of fisheries.

A Monastery could provide food for itself and a surplus for sale – even smaller establishments like Marrick Priory could sell barley and oats, although Marrick bought in wheat. The nuns there also sold hides, as did Selby Abbey, along with wool, pelts, and surplus tallow. The Bolton Priory canons did not seem to sell excess corn, but consumed it themselves, and money not needed to buy in extra during good years was used instead for luxuries.[13]

Consumption

Surviving accounts from Monasteries tend to come from the later period of their histories and indicate a move from the austere ideals of earlier times, but they also reflect the rise in living standards generally: the monks' way of life should be measured against what contemporary society came to expect as the norm.[14]

Consumption as revealed in the accounts should be related to the size of the Monastery. Attempts to estimate numbers in medieval households are based on an average amount of bread and ale considered necessary for one person. The Benedictine Rule said that a pound of bread a day and one 'hemina'[15] of wine or ale was sufficient. Ian Kershaw suggests that at Bolton Priory, where there were fewer than twenty canons and lay brothers, the establishment would have had over 200 people in all, including secular clerks, corrodians (permanent 'guests' of the abbey who had paid for their accommodation with a substantial gift to the Monastery), servants, hired workmen, and a changing number of visitors and supported paupers. Working from the total consumption of produce between 1305 and 1315, Kershaw estimates that one person had in a year 1,000 lb of grain as bread or pottage, 1,600 lb of malt made into ale,

160 lb of meat, and 25½ lb of butter and cheese. This works out at 19 lb of grain and over 3 lb of meat a week, but only about ½ lb of butter and cheese. Fruit and vegetable intake cannot be measured, but – as in medieval society as a whole – there may have been a vitamin C deficiency, especially in winter.[16] At Selby, the Pittancer's accounts (itemising the regular money allowance that was eventually made over to monks for the purchase of clothing and other personal necessities) reveal the number of monks at the Abbey each year: there were between 25 and 36 in the period 1412 to 1517, which compares with 70 monks at the larger Abbeys of Canterbury and Durham. Kershaw's method applied to the Selby Granger's account of 1404-5 gives a community of just over one hundred people. If Marrick Priory followed the 1440 Visitation regulations for Legbourne Priory in the Lincoln diocese, with one pound loaf and half a gallon of beer a day for the nuns, it had between 30 and 40 people in the year 1415-16.[17]

Monastic Diet Life for the monks was constrained by a Rule, whether derived from St Augustine, or St Benedict, or from various reformed and stricter versions. The Augustinians aimed for moderation, avoiding over-indulgence but realising that too much self-denial could affect the performance of a monk's duties.[18] The Benedictine Rule is the most well known. It was formulated at the beginning of the sixth century by St Benedict for a community at Monte Cassino in southern Italy, and was followed by the Benedictines, as at Selby, and more strictly by the reforming Cistercians. By the time of the Dissolution in England, it had been observed for 1,000 years, so obviously some changes must have been accepted. Apart from the changes in society, the geographical range of Monasteries has to be considered. The Rule stated that the only fire for heating should be in the warming house, and none made in the dormitory; but a building in southern Italy is not likely to be as cold as one in northern Europe.

The Measure of the Meat

St Benedict ordered the day around seven services, with Matins in the night. As the hours dividing the day were calculated from sunrise to sunset, their actual length varied, especially between winter and summer, and on the different latitudes, and it is difficult to fit these fluctuating 'hours' into the modern concept of a fixed 24-hour day. The most useful explanation is given by Louis J. Lekai in his book on the Cistercians:[19]

	June a.m.	December a.m.	
Rising	1.45	1.20	
MATINS	2.00	1.35	
End of Matins	3.00	2.25	
Interval			
LAUDS	3.10	7.00	Began at sunrise
Interval			Private masses
PRIME	4.00	8.00	
Chapter			In winter the
Work	5.00		sequence was
TERCE	7.45	9.20	Prime-mass-
Mass	8.00		Terce-Chapter
Reading	8.50		
SEXT	10.40	11.20	
		p.m.	
Dinner	11.00	1.35	
Siesta	p.m.		
NONE	2.00		In winter the
Work	2.30		None was said
VESPERS	6.00	3.30	before dinner
Supper	6.45		and dinner was
COMPLINE	7.30	4.00	followed by a
To bed	8.00	4.30	period of reading
			In winter there
			was no evening
			meal

This system gave six hours of manual work in summer but less than two in winter, when there was more reading and meditation. In midsummer the monks had less than six hours' sleep at night but had a rest at midday; in winter, when it was dark and cold, they had eight hours' sleep.

Hours of Meals

This seasonal division of the day makes sense of Chapter 41 of the Rule of St Benedict:

> From the feast of Easter until Pentecost let the brethren dine at the sixth hour and sup in the evening.
> From Pentecost throughout the summer . . . let them fast on Wednesdays and Fridays until the ninth hour; on other days let them dine at the sixth hour. If they have field work or the summer heat be extreme, this dinner at the sixth hour shall be the daily practice, according to the abbot's discretion . . .
> From September the 14th until the beginning of Lent let them always have their meal at the ninth hour.
> In Lent until Easter let them have it in the evening.
> Vespers, however, should be so timed that the brethren may not need lamplight at the meal, but that all may be accomplished by daylight.[20]

Modifications were made to this system. From the mid-ninth century, an extra drink was allowed, in the evening in winter or mid-afternoon in summer. On some days, this could be a finer wine accompanied by cakes or light bread. The evening drink took place in the refectory before the reading (*Collatio*) which preceded Compline. Also, varying from Monastery to Monastery, a second meal was eaten on certain days in winter.[21]

Measure of the Meat

The Rule of St Benedict

Chapter 39: The Measure of Food

We believe it to be sufficient for the daily meal . . . that every table should have two cooked dishes, on account of individual infirmities, so that he who perchance cannot eat of the one, may make his meal of the other . . . and if any fruit or young vegetables are available, let a third be added. Let a good pound weight of bread suffice for the day, whether there be one meal only, or both dinner and supper. But if their work chance to be heavier, the abbot shall have the choice and power, should it be expedient, to increase this allowance . . . Except the sick who are very weak, let all abstain from the flesh of four-footed animals.

Chapter 40: The Measure of Drink

Every man has his proper gift from God, one after this manner, and another after that. It is therefore with some misgiving that we determine how much others should eat and drink.

Nevertheless, keeping in view the needs of weaker brethren, we believe that a hemina of wine a day is sufficient for each. But those upon whom God bestows the gift of abstinence, should know that they shall have a special reward.

But if the circumstances of the place, or their work, or the heat of summer require more, let the superior be free to grant it.[22]

David Knowles says that the two cooked dishes were doubtless of flour, beans, eggs, cheese, etc., with fresh vegetables and fruit as available. He also assumes that earlier Anglo-Saxon Monasteries had beer, with wine more common after the Conquest.[23]

13

Later Benedictines fell short of the early ideals, prompting the formation of Cistercian Monasteries by reforming monks. Cîteaux itself was founded in 1098, and the first foundation in England was at Waverley in 1128. Rievaulx in Yorkshire was established in 1131, shortly followed by Fountains Abbey, which was founded by monks who left the Benedictine Abbey of St Mary, York, in 1132.[24] Aelred, who became third Abbot of Rievaulx in 1147, was immediately attracted to the Cistercian way of life when he first heard of it:

> By a happy chance he heard tell, from a close friend of his, how, two years or more before, certain monks had come to England from across the sea, wonderful men, famous adepts in the religious life, white monks by name and white also in vesture. For their name arose from the fact that, as the angels might be, they were clothed in undyed wool spun and woven from the pure fleece of the sheep . . . For them everything is fixed by weight, measure and number. A pound of bread, a pint[25] of drink, two dishes of cabbage and beans. If they sup, the remnants of their former meal are dished up again except that, instead of two cooked dishes, fresh vegetables, if they are to be had, are served.[26]

In other words, the Cistercians in 1134 were following the precise instructions of St Benedict's Rule laid down in the early sixth century.

There are many examples of Monasteries failing in this ideal. Even the less strict Augustinians had to have their moderation enforced at times. The Visitation of Archbishop Wickwane to Bolton Priory in 1280 found the canons eating too sumptuous meals, and drinking after Compline.[27] The ideal was self-discipline through abstinence, as the Rule of St Benedict expressed:

The Measure of the Meat

Chapter 49: Of the Observance of Lent
The Life of a monk ought at all times to be
lenten in character; but since few have the
strength for that, we therefore urge that in these
days of Lent the brethren should lead lives of great
purity . . . let us add something beyond the wonted
measure of our service, such as private prayers and
abstinence in food and drink.[28]

Eating of Meat

The monks' diet was not 'vegetarian' in the modern sense,
but they denied themselves meat as a form of self-discipline.
Benedict had required abstinence only from four-footed
animals, so presumably the flesh of birds could have been
eaten, but this does not seem to be mentioned particularly.
Fish was the common alternative in medieval society during
Lent and other fast days. Some of the stricter Orders seem
to have been completely vegetarian, but by the end of the
twelfth century fish was allowed on certain occasions,
probably because it was necessary to provide a reasonable
diet.[29] Fish was not allowed for the Cistercians, except for
the sick, until the thirteenth century, after which they
developed fish farming on a large scale. Waverley Abbey
was granted land for a fish pond in 1250, and it has been
suggested that this reflected the new dispensation.[30]
In a tenth-century *Colloquium* by the Anglo-Saxon
Aelfric, there is a conversation between a pupil in a
Monastery and his master: the boy says he eats vegetables,
eggs, fish, cheese, butter, and beans, as well as the meat he
is allowed because he is young.[31] This suggests that the
monks were allowed to eat fish, and it is only meat that
differentiates the boy's diet.
Apart from the exemption of children being educated in
the Monasteries, there were other relaxations to the Rule
forbidding meat, all occurring outside the Refectory. The
Abbot's duties included the entertainment of important

guests, and to prevent disruption to the monastic routine he had his own kitchen to cater for these, in which meat could be prepared.[32] He was permitted to break his own fast to join his guests if he wished. Meat was also allowed to the sick in the Infirmary, including those monks undergoing the periodic bloodletting, and food was prepared for them in a separate kitchen. When monks were allowed to have meat on certain occasions, they ate in a separate room from the normal Refectory, called the Misericord.[33] Probably because the Infirmary already catered for a meat diet, this Misericord was often built on to the Infirmary, as at Waverley and Fountains.

Generally, abstinence from meat is thought to have been the Rule in England during the tenth, eleventh, and early twelfth centuries. The Augustinians may not have practised total abstinence, arguing that the fault 'lay not in tasting but in desiring, not in food but in greed'. Gerald of Wales (late twelfth to early thirteenth centuries) said that the regular canons ate meat 'three days in the week; on the other days they eat fish, eggs and cheese in the refectory'.[34] The canons at Bolton Priory were certainly eating meat by the end of the thirteenth century, when two-thirds of their expenditure was on fish and a third on meat; by 1320 expenditure was at least equal. The Benedictines were in due course allowed meat on Sundays, Mondays, Tuesdays, and Thursdays, except in Advent and Lent; and eating meat was certainly accepted by 1421, when the Benedictines were discussing reform.[35]

The Cistercians took longer to make the change; in the mid-thirteenth century they were still eating only fish and eggs themselves whilst providing meat only for servants.[36] In 1256 there was no alteration of the Rule noted in the General Chapter, but the early fourteenth century saw dispensations if they had difficulty obtaining vegetables. In 1335 they could eat meat in the Infirmary, or by invitation at the Abbot's table. Eating in the Infirmary must have become popular, because a decree of 1439 said that no one was to eat there more than twice a week, and at least two-thirds of the community had to be eating in the Refectory at any one time. In 1486, after a request to the Pope, the new observance was formally allowed, and meat could be eaten on Sundays, Tuesdays, and Thursdays.[37] These decisions must have recognised what was already happening, for Abbots had the power to make decisions based on circumstances, and diet suitable for a Monastery in southern Italy, where St Benedict formulated his Rule, could not always be applied successfully in a monastery in northern England.

Food and Feast

Analysis of the Bolton Priory accounts of 1305–15 indicates that the staple diet was based on grain and ale, and that if the monks had the fresh vegetables and fruit recommended in Benedict's diet, these would have come from home produce and would not be reflected in the accounts. The Benedictine Rule allowed two dishes to be offered, so that there was a choice, giving opportunity for individual abstinences and acknowledging personal taste. Nevertheless, there were further opportunities for variety in diet, apart from that offered in the Infirmary. The Abbot entertained important visitors to the Monastery; but if he were not entertaining he could invite some of the monks to dine with him, and presumably they benefited from the relaxed regime of his kitchen.[38]

There were also specific breakfasts on certain days. The Sacrist at Marrick Priory paid 4s 9d for the Convent's breakfast on Easter morning in 1416, and the Selby Sacrist gave the customary breakfast to the priests on Easter day 1447.[39] Saint's days and anniversaries gave an excuse for a special dish. The money allowance or pittance (derived from the same word as piety) originally came from the bequests of money made in order to have mass said for the donor's soul, and it was used to provide something extra for the monk (although later the term was extended to mean the personal and clothing allowance of each monk).[40] This treat could be a special dish of fish, or the provision of a more delicate white bread (pandemain). The feasts on special occasions could be elaborate. Gerald of Wales described a Trinity Sunday dinner at Christ Church, Canterbury, at the end of the twelfth century; he 'counted sixteen courses, cooked in the most exquisite manner; delicacies were also sent down by the prior from the high table to individuals'.[41] Such feasts may have been the occasions when musicians were paid for their services in the Selby Bursars' account of 1398–9: they appear several times in December, as well as at Easter and the Ascension. Waferers were also paid, including on 6 October, the Feast of the Burial of St Germain, patron saint of the Abbey.[42] Wafers were a kind of light biscuit, cooked on special wafering irons, but they could be presented in elaborate confections that would provide a fitting end to a feast.

Even if the monks were abstaining from meat, they did not have to abstain from variety in a feast. The religious men attending the funeral feast of Nicholas Bubwyth, Bishop of Bath and Wells, on 4 December 1424, had as much choice as did the others, with special fish versions of the items on the menu (see Appendix).

Charity

Monastic charity supported a number of paupers. The canons at Waltham Abbey were allowed a large daily diet, but they each supported at least one destitute man. Bolton Priory gave corn, sometimes mixed with oatmeal, and beans in alms; during 1298–1304, just over 190 quarters of corn were given to the poor.[43]

Selby Abbey's charity is revealed through the Granger's and Almoner's accounts. In 1404–05, 4 quarters of wheat were given to mendicant friars, and 2 quarters 4 bushels of wheat were used for bread to be distributed to the poor on Maundy Thursday; it was noted that wheat had to be used that year because of the poor quality of rye. The bulk of wheat was kept for the Abbey's own use; but it was more

18

generous with beans and peas. The Abbey itself used 13 quarters, whilst 5 quarters 6 bushels went in alms; 21 quarters were used for horse fodder. The Almoner in 1434–5 made gifts of clothing and fuel to three poor people; he also purchased 6 quarters of rye to distribute to the poor on Abbey festivals, along with a small amount of pork and beef, and 1,000 red herrings.[44]

The Granger at Marrick Priory also accounted for alms during the year 1415–16. Three bushels of peas were given in alms on the feast day of the patron saint, Andrew, which compares well with the total of 3 bushels used for pottage by the Priory that year. Meanwhile, 4 bushels were used for pig food.[45]

It seems clear that the poor were given what was considered a lesser grain, also used for animal fodder, and not consumed in large quantities by the monks or nuns themselves. However, food passed on to the poor from the Refectory itself is not accounted for, and a monk could have the chance of making charitable gifts through his own abstinence.

The Monastic Household

A Monastery was organised in very much the same way as other large medieval households. The Abbot may have had important family connections and have been accorded respect in his own right, but he also represented the Monastery as a wealthy landowner with economic power. His establishment was separately financed at Selby Abbey, with the oversight of the Bursar's office. Other activities in the Monastery had their own office and finances, just as in secular households. The monks took it in turns to hold the position of accountant for a year, and at the end produced their accounts, a few of which have survived. The two Bursars, Cellarer, Granger, Kitchener, Refectorer, and others left records of their expenditure, although unfortunately they are not complete for Selby, and a survey of all the offices in any one year is not possible.

The Rule of St Benedict, Chapters 35 and 46, arranged

for the monks or nuns to take it in turns to work in the kitchen, cellar, bakehouse, brewhouse, or vegetable garden, so that they all served one another. This service was usually undertaken for a week, and took the form of practical help rather than the financial accounting of the office-holders. At the end of the week, there would be a formal handing over of equipment to the next incumbents. In the kitchen the old server would wash all the towels, and he and the new server would wash the feet of all the other monks.[46]

The accounts and occasional inventories help to give a picture of the offices and their furnishings. At the Dissolution in 1539, Bolton Priory had pewter and brass vessels, and iron and wooden implements in the kitchen; with other equipment in the larderhouse, flesh larderhouse, malthouse, brewery, cellar, and Refectory. The small Nunnery at Esholt had in its cellar in 1360 three maplewood goblets (mazers), seven silver spoons, three casks of ale, and three poorer casks of ale, two small trestle tables, two balances, and one salting cloth; and the bakehouse had a lead vat in the baking oven and three portable lead vats. Its kitchen had seven brass pots, four posnets, four large pans and three smaller pans. The Dissolution Visitation of Esholt Priory found 'a kychyn of the olde ffasshyon w^t ane vpright roofe after the ffasshyon of a louer, and hath a range conteynyng in length xij ffoote, and in the same kychyn ij ffayre ovens, wherof they may bake in th'one a quarter and in th'other half a quarter'. Selby's kitchen had a high lantern with eight corners, which was releaded in 1398–9 at the Bursar's expense; it had a weathercock on top.[47]

The Selby Kitchener oversaw the preparation of food for the monks' table, and the maintenance of the equipment and kitchen. The account of 1416–17 provides many details. An ash tree was felled and squared to be used as a dresser; eighty wooden dishes, plates, and saucers were purchased, along with two earthenware jars, two strainers, a brass ladle, a basket for carrying turves, and two hampers for the poulterer. A knife for dressing meat and a 'lechingknyf' (slicing knife) were bought from Robert Smith, who also repaired two 'skoinours' (perhaps skimmers) and other faulty utensils, and made a hasp and staple for the vat used for soaking fish. William Plummer repaired lead vessels, and Nicholas Couper provided new hoops for vats. The mustard-grinding stones were mended, and Roger Cooke repaired the ranges in the kitchen. Charcoal for use in the kitchen was made in the woods at Hambleton.[48]

The Abbot of Selby had his own cook. In 1398–9 this office was held at first by Henry Droury, who died during that year, when John Hasand took over. His wage was 20*s* a year, and he was assisted by two pages, a servant in the storehouse, and a servant in the guesthouse, who all received salaries. The Monastery kitchen had another cook, also paid 20*s* a year. In 1416–17, he was John Barley, aided by the poulterer William Pinne, the scullion Thomas Ripon, and three pages, Robert Bernard, Robert de Aland, and Robert Maunsell. Agnes Bernard was the 'preparer of animal intestines', and received a salary of 6*s* 8*d*. Marrick Priory also employed a cook, John in 1415–16, who received 12*s*. He was assisted by two maids of the bakehouse and storeroom, and a kitchen maid.[49]

It is important to note that these were professional cooks,[50] not to be confused with the monks, who were referred to as 'Brother' in the accounts. They had their own permanent servants to assist them, in addition to any help in taking food to the refectory that would have been given by the weekly servers. The popular picture of monks scurrying around a kitchen doing the cooking cannot be sustained, certainly not by the fifteenth century.

The Refectory, where the kitchen's produce was eaten, was supposed to be a quiet place. Benedict's Rule said the only voice to be heard should be that of the reader. The servers, who had been allowed a drink and some bread before going on duty, were to see to the needs of the diners, who could communicate their needs by use of signs. Towels would be put out at the laver in the cloister, and tablecloths and napkins provided. Cloths were also laid on the cupboards, on which cups and vessels – such as the mazers known at Esholt and Selby – would be set out. At Selby, the Refectorer also provided reed mats for the benches.[51]

The Cistercians were known for their good table manners. They had to hold their drinking cups in both hands, reach out for the salt with the tip of their knives, and wipe the used plates with a piece of bread, not their napkins.[52] Monastic table manners were appreciated in society, and Chaucer's Prioress provides an example.

Food The limited numbers of examples cited here can give insight into the self-sufficiency of the monasteries and the proportions of different items of food eaten.

Grain

Wheat was the most desired crop. Esholt Priory grew some and received some as tithes, but had to buy in most of what it needed in the period 1360–5. Marrick Priory bought 79 quarters 5 bushels of wheat and maslin (mixed wheat and rye) in 1415–16, and used 70 quarters of this for baking bread on twenty-six occasions, which suggests one baking session a fortnight. Most of the rest went in allowances to servants and the poor. The Selby Granger accounted for 412 quarters in 1404–05, including some received as payment of rents.[53]

Oats were a northern crop, easier to grow than wheat. In 1360–5 Esholt grew 66 acres of oats, compared with 14 of wheat and 12½ of rye, and Marrick had 102 quarters of oats in its own cultivation in 1415–16. Marrick used 48 quarters of oats for wort in brewing, 10 quarters for (presumably) pottage, and 17 quarters for horse and pig fodder. Bolton Priory in 1296–8 had 100 quarters of oatmeal, used for pottage, about half the amount of wheat they used for bread. In 1404–05, the Selby Granger accounted for 24 quarters of oatmeal for pottage, 180 quarters for malt (mixed with barley and dredge – dredge itself was oats and barley sown together), and 168 quarters for horse fodder, feeding the hunting dogs of the warren, and fattening the swans in the dam and ditches of the Abbey, the peacocks and capons. He used a far greater amount of dredge and barley for wort, the unfermented infusion of malt.[54]

Only a small proportion of oats was used for the monks' and nuns' pottage; most went for brewing, and for horse fodder, dog food, and fattening pigs and birds. Monks and nuns seem to have been of a social status that expected wheat bread, with the superior pandemain for the Abbot and his guests, and for the monks on special occasions. Lesser grain was used for servants' allowances and for charity. The Sacrist at Selby in 1446–7 bought 4,000 obleys (wafers) in York, whilst Marrick Priory baked its own obleys.[55] Only the Carthusians, as part of their more austere regime, were given rye bread. Even the Cistercians had wheat bread, according to a story from the mid-thirteenth century, when a prospective lay brother gave as his reason for wishing to join: 'white bread and often'.[56]

Meat and Fish

All the accounts examined here come from a period after meat became an acceptable part of the diet; and it formed a large part of what was consumed. The earliest accounts are those of 1287–1319 at Bolton Priory, analysed by Ian Kershaw. They illustrate a period when the new diet was becoming established, and show a growth in meat purchases over fish. Through the years 1304–15, they slaughtered an average of 98 cattle (oxen, cows, and a few young cattle), 122 sheep, and 93 pigs a year. At Selby, the Extern Cellarer in 1413 accounted for animals he bought (as opposed to existing stock); these included three bullocks 'for fattening towards the festival of Easter' and forty-eight bullocks during the rest of the year. Other references already cited show that the Abbey kept a rabbit warren with hunting dogs, and fattened swans, pigeons, capons, and peacocks. The Selby

Kitchener's account of 1416–17 itemises a whole range of food consumed 'by the lord abbot, convent and other visitors' in the year, and is thus an extremely interesting source of information about the monks' diet. They had 100 beef animals (half were cows, the rest oxen, bullocks, or calves, with one heifer); 76 pigs, 28 piglets, and 3 boars; 383 sheep and 66 lambs; 45 coneys and rabbits; 8 swans and cygnets; 26 geese, 71 ducks, 36 capons, 100 cocks and hens, 24 chickens, 731 pigeons, 18 partridges, 2 pheasants, and 24 herons. Two further pigs were diseased and 'of no use for consumption', and ten sheep had been torn apart by the dogs of the rabbit warren.[57]

The Selby Kitchener also meticulously noted the amount of fish, which came from the fishery belonging to his office, the Abbot's fishery at Crowle in Lincolnshire, and the dam at Selby; his expenses included a trammel net bought 'for taking fish in the dam'. He also bought dried and salted fish, and some salmon, from Scarborough, Hull, and York. The total consumed by the Monastery and its guests in 1416–17 was: 38,590 red herrings, with 1,200 more going to the poor on Maundy Thursday and 112 on All Saints Day; 1,440 white herrings; 474 salted fish; 869 dried fish – no doubt soaked in the vat that was given a new hasp and staple that year; 104½ salmon, 2½ sprents or young salmon and 1 'cokke'; 5 great eels from Crowle, and 1,216 smaller eels from Crowle and the Selby dam; 1 tench, 12 pikes, 67 pickerels, and 4,440 roach and perch from Crowle and Selby.[58]

Dairy Produce and Eggs

Only a relatively small proportion of dairy produce seems to have been included in the monks' diet, although the true amount may be hidden as it was home produced and not accounted for. In 1380 Esholt spent 3s 4d on dairy produce, compared with 13s 4d on 'meats received' and 6s 8d on salt. Out of a total of £33 1s 2½d in 1415–16, Marrick Priory spent £2 5s 3d on butter and eggs and 2s 11d on cheese:

most of their costs were for grain. Bolton Priory's average consumption between 1305 and 1315 has been assessed at only 25½ lb of butter and cheese per person a year. In 1416–17 Selby used 2,240 eggs, and a further 400 were 'thrown out because bad'; 173 gallons of milk and 7½ stones of cheese came from the Abbey's dairy at nearby Stainer. Two earthenware jars to carry milk were bought in the same year.[59]

Beans and Peas

Beans and peas were both used for pottage. In 1398–9 the Bursars of Selby bought 3 quarters of beans and 3 quarters and 4 bushels of green peas for this purpose, and the Granger in 1404–05 bought 3 quarters of green peas. The Kitchener of 1416–17 used 3 quarters and 5 bushels 'for making pottage with' for the Abbot and convent, with a further 1 quarter 1 bushel during Lent; a far greater amount, 12 quarters, went 'in feeding and sustenance of pigs'. This can be compared with Marrick Priory in 1415–16, which used 3 bushels for pottage, 4 bushels in alms on the festival of St Andrew, and 4 bushels for pig food.[60] Peas were thus another crop given more readily to the poor and used for animal fodder rather than eaten by monks and nuns.

Vegetables

Fresh vegetables and fruits are a hidden item, because they were grown domestically and not accounted for. However, the Bursar at Marrick in 1415–16 paid for the repair of the walls of the cabbage garden – 'del kalgarth wall'. In 1416–17, the Selby Kitchener bought cabbage, leeks, garlic, and onions, but he did not itemise their use. He also paid Roger Cooke (who had repaired the ranges in the kitchen) for 'digging in the garden called Herynghousgarth for 3 days in order to plant and sow herbs there'.[61]

Spices and Other Items

Between 1287 and 1319 Bolton Priory bought pepper,

saffron, cummin, mace, and cloves, together with rice, sugar, raisins, almonds, and figs.[62] These are all typical ingredients of medieval cuisine revealed in contemporary recipes, when a sharp taste in spices was preferred (rather than the cinnamon and ginger more dominant in sixteenth-century recipes), and dried fruit and sugar were added to meat dishes. Saffron was popular, used for colour as much as taste. Almonds were a major item, especially ground and mixed with a liquid to replace milk during Lent and fast days.

Betwen 1360 and 1365 Esholt Priory only specified salt, which cost 6s 8d, but spices may have been included under 'other things'. Marrick spent 23s 4d on salt in 1415–16, and 15d on pepper and saffron.[63]

The Selby accounts again give us a more detailed picture. In 1398–9 the Bursars made three purchases of spices for the Abbot, not described but totalling £9 1s 1d. They also bought green ginger from Hull, more green ginger about St Valentine's Day (costing 3s 4d), and a measure of figs and raisins at 8s. Further items may have been among the 'victuals' bought by the Abbot's cooks. The Kitchener's account for 1416–17 lists the purchase of spices, which were all used 'in victuals of the lord abbot, the convent, and other visitors this year': 17 quarters and 4 bushels of salt at £3 8s 4d; 19 lb of pepper at £1 15s; 5¼ lb of saffron at £2 15s 3d (then, as now, the most expensive item for its weight); 98 lb of almonds at £1 3s 3d; 113½ lb of rice at 11s 9½d; 2 lb of sanders (used to colour food red) at 2s 5d; 2 lb of cummin at 4d; 13 lb of figs at 13d and a measure of figs and raisins at 15s; and 20 gallons and 1 pottle of honey at 17s 1d. Mustard (2 bushels and 3 pecks), lard (48½ lb) and oil (7¼ gallons) were listed under 'Small expenses'.[64]

Ale and Wine

In the English Monasteries noted here, ale was the staple drink, with a large proportion of barley and oats diverted to the production of malt. The office of Granger at Selby

Abbey included the oversight of both the bakehouse and brewhouse, and wages were paid to the baker, the brewer and their assistants. Repairs were needed to the gylefat (vat for fermenting alewort) and other vessels and casks in 1404–05, as well as to the malt room and malthouse. Loss of malt in the process of malting had to be noted, as well as 'destruction by worms called weevils', and by rats and mice. A total of 752 quarters of malt were delivered for brewing ale on fifty-two occasions, which suggests the Abbey brewed once a week. In 1416–17 the Kitchener received 625 quarters of malt 'brewed for consumption by the lord Abbot, convent and other visitors this year'.[65]

In 1307–08, Bolton Priory had three brewings a fortnight, to produce 2,000 gallons of ale. Marrick had 84 quarters of malt delivered to the Convent brewery on thirteen occasions during 1415–16, suggesting one brewing a month.[66]

Wine at Selby was bought by the Bursars for the Abbot and his guests, but there is no indication from the accounts that it was used in the Monastery kitchen. The Extern Cellarer's accounts show it was bought for refreshment during official business, and it appears in the Sacrist's account of 1446–7 as a communion wine.[67]

Sources of Supplies

From 1298 Bolton Priory purchased cloth, fish, spices, and other foodstuffs from St Botolph's Fair in Lincolnshire. Selby Abbey purchased from Selby and the surrounding area, and it had its own estates. Supplies also came from York, Scarborough, Hull, Pontefract, and Howden, and the Kitchener bought pepper in London. These were transported by horse – there are expenses for saddles, girths, saddle pads, and a halter, with the costs of shoeing – and carried in baskets and hampers, with earthenware jars to bring milk from Stainer. Because Selby was on the River Ouse, water transport was also possible.[68]

The Monastery Building Evidence for monastic diet can be assembled from documentary sources, but can also be seen in more tangible form. Surviving sites throughout the country reveal through the remains of church, cloister, and chapter house the spiritual function of the Monasteries, whilst the household arrangements can be seen in the Abbot's quarters, Refectory, and kitchens, Infirmary and guest house, as well as the associated bakehouse, brewhouse, storerooms, barns, and stables.

Esholt and Marrick Priories

The smaller establishments seem closest to the typical domestic plan. Nothing now remains of Esholt Priory, apart from a few stones incorporated into the eighteenth-century Esholt Hall, but a detailed description in the Dissolution Survey enables an impression of the Nunnery to be gained. It had the traditional cloister, with church on the north and chapterhouse on the east; and to the south, on a north–south axis, was a hall with screens passage at the south end, and associated buttery, pantry, and parlour beyond. A larder house, malt chamber, and brewhouse were nearby, and the kitchen, probably separate, was 'of the olde ffasshyon'. The site also included barns, ox, cow, and swine houses, stables and carthouse, stores for wood and coal, and a close and orchards. There were several parlours, including one off the cloister with a fireplace and glazed bay windows, and three at the south end of the nuns' dorter, 'callid the ladyes parlers', all with glass windows, two with fireplaces, and one with a kitchen attached.[69]

This domestic cosiness may have been more typical of the smaller Nunneries. A similar plan can be discerned at Marrick. After the Dissolution, it was acquired by John Ulvedale, one of the Commissioners of Suppression. In 1549 it passed to his son Avery, who in turn bequeathed it to his son John. In 1588 it was bought by Richard Brackenbury of London, and then in 1592 by Timothy Hutton of Bishop Auckland. A plan of the Priory may relate to this change of ownership.[70] It shows the buildings already in domestic use – 'stable for my owne geldinges' must be from this later ownership – but the memory of the Nunnery, with its cloister, dorter, nuns' court, and chamber of the Prioress, is still strong. The associated offices of milkhouse, bakehouse, brew house, kiln and storehouses could be those also used by the nuns, together with stables, oxhouse, dovehouse, and even slaughterhouse. Dog kennels may have been added by a later owner, but it should be remembered that Selby Abbey was not unusual in keeping a dog pack: so also did Chaucer's Prioress. The kitchen, screens passage, and hall lie on an east–west axis to the south of the cloister, with a parlour beyond. The nuns also had two little gardens and an orchard within their Convent walls.

The larger Abbeys lose this more domestic order of kitchen, screens passage, and hall, although the Refectory and kitchen are usually found to the south of the cloister.

Kirkstall Abbey

The Cistercians especially built to a common plan, from their first English Monastery at Waverley[71] to the several Yorkshire houses. Kirkstall Abbey is taken as the example here, and it provides interesting information for a study of monastic eating habits.

The site at Kirkstall seems to have been inhabited by hermits when Abbot Alexander chanced upon it and acquired it for his Cistercian monks who were finding life uncongenial at Barnoldswick. Construction of the Abbey was begun in 1152, and the main buildings were completed by the time of Alexander's death in 1182. The Infirmary was added in the early 1200s, followed by the Abbot's house about 1230. Later came the guest house, to the west of the church, and the ground plan of its hall, pantry, buttery, and kitchen has been revealed in excavation. All these additions had their own kitchens.[72]

The Refectory and kitchens at Kirkstall were along the south side of the cloister. W. H. St John Hope had argued

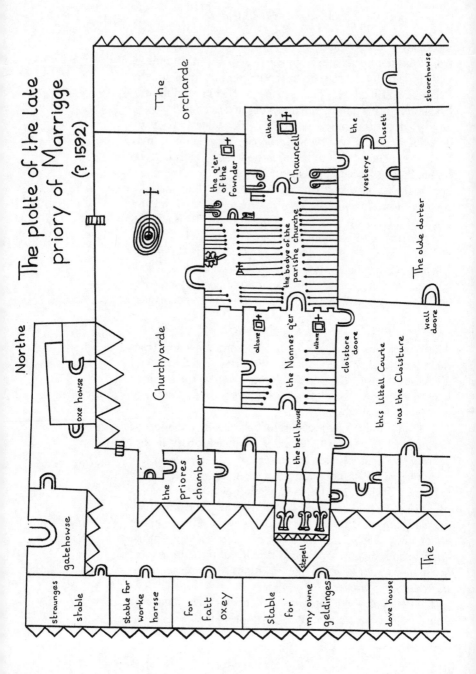

The plotte of the late priory of Marrigge (? 1592)

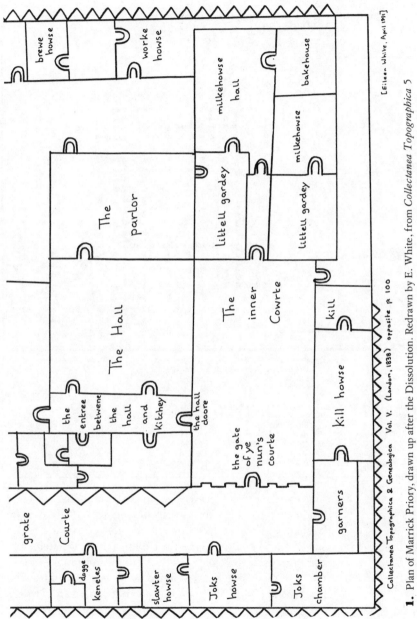

1. Plan of Marrick Priory, drawn up after the Dissolution. Redrawn by E. White, from *Collectanea Topographica 5* (1838), facing p. 100.

The labels within the plan, as drawn:

brewe howse

worke howse

milkehouse hall

bakehouse

The parlor

littell gardey

milkehouse

littell gardey

The Hall

The inner Cowrte

kill

the entree betwene the hall and kitchey

the hall doore

kill howse

the gate of ye nun's cowrte

grate Cowrte

dogge keneles

slawter howse

Joks howse

Joks chamber

garners

[Eileen White 1991]

Collectanea Topographica & Genealogica Vol. V. (London, 1838) opposite p. 100

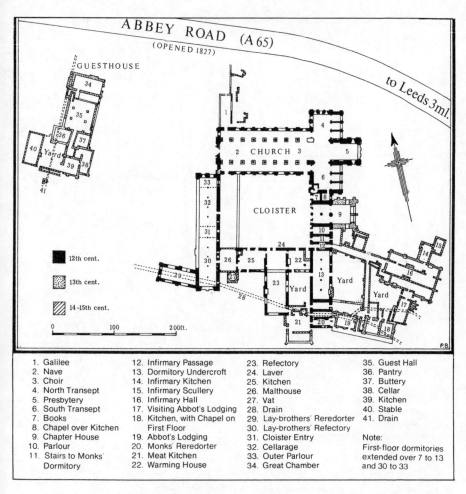

ABBEY ROAD (A 65)
(OPENED 1827)

to Leeds 3ml.

GUESTHOUSE

CHURCH

CLOISTER

12th cent.

13th cent.

14-15th cent.

0   100   200ft.

Yard

Yard

Yard

P.B.

1.	Galilee	12.	Infirmary Passage	23.	Refectory	35.	Guest Hall
2.	Nave	13.	Dormitory Undercroft	24.	Laver	36.	Pantry
3.	Choir	14.	Infirmary Kitchen	25.	Kitchen	37.	Buttery
4.	North Transept	15.	Infirmary Scullery	26.	Malthouse	38.	Cellar
5.	Presbytery	16.	Infirmary Hall	27.	Vat	39.	Kitchen
6.	South Transept	17.	Visiting Abbot's Lodging	28.	Drain	40.	Stable
7.	Books	18.	Kitchen, with Chapel on	29.	Lay-brothers' Reredorter	41.	Drain
8.	Chapel over Kitchen		First Floor	30.	Lay-brothers' Refectory		
9.	Chapter House	19.	Abbot's Lodging	31.	Cloister Entry		Note:
10.	Parlour	20.	Monks' Reredorter	32.	Cellarage		First-floor dormitories
11.	Stairs to Monks'	21.	Meat Kitchen	33.	Outer Parlour		extended over 7 to 13
	Dormitory	22.	Warming House	34.	Great Chamber		and 30 to 33

2.

Plan of Kirkstall
Abbey by P. Brears.

that the first Refectory lay on an east–west line; this was vindicated in the excavations during the 1950s.[73] The kitchen was at the west end of the Refectory, and had a small central hearth. In the thirteenth century the Refectory was enlarged, presumably because there were more monks to accommodate. It was realigned north–south, towards the river bank, and the kitchen was extended eastwards, with a new double hearth in its centre; the two hearths placed back to back and facing east and west. A new building was attached to its south side, possibly a scullery. The lay brothers had their own Refectory and dorter on the west side of the cloister, but were provided with food from the choir monks' kitchen; the serving hatch from their Refectory to the covered lane between that and the kitchen remains. This arrangement continued for about two hundred years.

In the later fifteenth century, judging from the style of architecture employed in the reconstruction, the Refectory was divided into two storeys; the original high windows were blocked and new ones created in the current style. The pulpitum on the west side, from which a monk had read to the diners below, and the stairs leading to it inside the thickness of the wall, were filled in, and a new fireplace was added. Alterations were made along the cloister wall, so that the upper storey could be reached through one doorway and a staircase, and the lower Refectory entered through another door to the east.[74] These alterations reflect the fact that by 1450 the Cistercians were allowed to eat meat on certain days, as long as it was in a separate Refectory or Misericord. In some Monasteries, such as Waverley or Fountains, the architectural evidence suggests that the Misericord was attached to the Infirmary hall, a logical arrangement as the Infirmary kitchen already had dispensation to serve meat to the patients. At Kirkstall, the other solution was adopted, and the Refectory itself was divided, with two entrances. The upper storey continued to be served from the original kitchen, and the ground floor was the Misericord. It had a border of broad flagstones, on which the tables would be set up, and a central area of inlaid tiles, red, yellow, and blue, set in a pattern; these had obviously been relaid, as they are thirteenth century in style. Serving the Misericord was a new meat kitchen, built to the south of the warming house yard attached to the south-east corner of the Refectory. There were two fireplaces on the north and west sides, with a small oven connected to

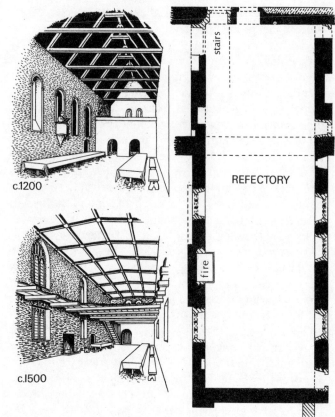

3.
The Refectory at
Kirkstall Abbey.
Drawing by
P. Brears.

the left of the northern fireplace, its base still preserved, and a larger independent oven to the right of this fireplace, projecting into the yard on the north. The remains of a smaller hearth were found in the centre of the room. On the south side were three rooms, the central one with a floor of stone slabs with mortared edges which could have been a meat store. The western room had a flagged floor with a trough or sink discharging to a drain, which may have been a scullery.[75]

By this time, there were no lay brothers, and their former

34

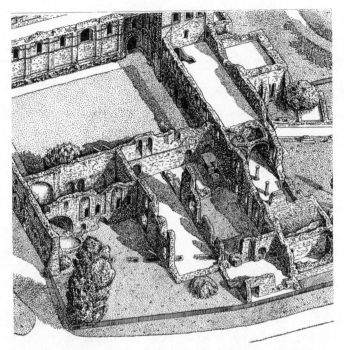

4.
The ruins of
Kirkstall Abbey
showing the
buildings south of
the cloister: the
kitchen (left), the
Refectory and the
later meat kitchen
(lower right).
Drawing by
P. Brears.

quarters did not need a Misericord added.[76] The original
kitchen continued to serve the upper Refectory, but at some
time it was used temporarily for bronze-casting (repair
work, or for a new bell); when it was reconverted to a
kitchen it had a smaller hearth and a new flagged floor.[77]
The original lay brothers' passage, along the west side of the
cloister, and leading south between the lay brothers' quarters
and the kitchen, had been blocked off long before; in the
final period of the Abbey's existence, this area seems to
have become a malthouse and bakehouse. An oven was
built into the west kitchen wall from the enclosed passage,
and a large vat constructed to the south, the foundations of
which are still visible, and which meant the destruction of
the scullery once built onto the kitchen. Coal and charcoal
fragments were found in the yard south of the kitchen. By

the Dissolution, there were only thirty monks, and the large double fireplace of earlier centuries may have been unnecessary.

Remains of shellfish, mostly oysters but also mussels, cockles, and whelks, had been found associated with this kitchen, but the 1956 and 1957 excavations unearthed a larger dump of animal bones to the south-west of the meat kitchen. The area covered about 25 by 40 yards, and was 18 inches to 3 feet deep. At first it was thought that rubbish had been brought from another site to fill in the uneven hollows of the ground, as soil, stones, and pottery fragments were included. Later, it was considered to be an original dump, with bones and other rubbish being covered by a layer of soil as they were deposited. The dump may have been begun before the meat kitchen was built, as part of the scullery drain lay over the lowest layer, perhaps when there was a temporary timber meat kitchen in use. The bones of about 5,000 animals were found, accumulating over the last fifty years of the Monastery's existence. About 90 per cent of them came from ox, 5 per cent from sheep (two breeds were identified), 3 per cent from pigs, and 2 per cent from deer (red, roe, and fallow deer).[78] Other bones were of goat, rabbit, hare, domestic fowl, duck, geese, pigeons, heron, woodcock, blackcock, and large fish that could have been cod or salmon.

The meat came from mature animals, probably draught oxen too old to work, at 5–10 years, and dairy cows; the sheep were about 2–3 years old; and the pigs 18 months. Most of the bones were chopped, and some chopped a second time, suggesting the meat was stewed, not roasted: the only way to cook the meat of draught oxen.

Just south of the Refectory and meat kitchen was a circular building, now gone but visible on a 1723 engraving by Samuel Buck, considered to be a dovecot, and a reminder that Monasteries, like manors, were allowed the privilege of erecting them.[79] A series of buildings and walls in the same area, some probably demolished when the meat kitchen was built, may mark the site of vegetable gardens and orchards on the land reclaimed from the River Aire. An old course of the river, closer to the Abbey than the present line, may have been sealed off by dumping soil in the early thirteenth century, to create a series of fishponds, two of which survived to the eighteenth century. Part of a jetty or edge of a pond was found south of the Refectory, thought to date from the later twelfth century. If a fishpond were such an early feature, then it may have been used for the Infirmary kitchen, for Cistercians were not even allowed fish until later in the thirteenth century, although it should be considered that practice, especially in Monasteries in a northern climate, could have preceded official sanction. The excavations in the 1950s do not seem to have found or identified large amounts of freshwater fish bones.[80]

Conclusion

The archways leading to the chapter house on the east side of the cloister at Kirkstall can still be admired, demonstrating one of the major decorative features allowed in Cistercian architecture. The wall along the south side is no less interesting, with arches marking the lavatorium, where the monks could wash their hands before entering the Refectory. The wall also shows signs of the alterations that went on behind it to the warming house, Refectory, and kitchen, reflecting how changes to the monastic diet can be embodied in a permanent architectural record.

The evidence from only a few Monasteries has raised some interesting points which could be enhanced by similar examination of material from elsewhere. Detailed work could perhaps indicate when meat-eating became accepted by the different Orders.

It is clear that whereas monks may not have escaped deprivation caused by poor harvests, and may have had a strict imposition of Lenten diet, or imposed it on themselves, they could draw on the produce of extensive property, and usually expected food reflecting their status in society. In the context of medieval life, they did not fare badly.

Appendix A menu showing how a religious diet was catered for at a feast:

> *Conuiuium domini Nicholai Bubbewyth, nuper episcopi Bathonensis & Wellensis ad funeralia; videlicet, quarto die decembris, anno domini Millesimo. CCCC^{mo} vecessimo quarto:*
> (Feast at the funeral of the lord Nicholas Bubbewyth, late bishop of Bath and Wells; that is to say on 4 December 1424)

in carnibus (in meat)	*Conuiuium de piscibus pro viris* *Religiosis ad funeralia predicta* (Fish feast for the religious men at the said funeral)
Le .j. cours	Le .j. cours
Nomblys de Roo	Elys in sorry
Blamangere	Blamanger
Braun, cum Mustard	Bakoun heryng
Chynes de porke	Mulwyl taylys
Capoun Roste de	Lenge taylys
haut grece	
Swan Roste	Jollys of Samoun
Heroun Rostyd	Merlyng sode
Aloes de Roo	Pyke
Puddyng de Swan necke	Grete Plays
Vn Lechemete	Leche barry
Vn bake, *videlicet*	Crustade Ryal
Crustade	
Le .ij. cours	Le .ij. cours
Ro Styuyd	
Mammenye	Mammenye
Connyng Rostyd	Crem of Almaundys
Curlew	Codelyng
Fesaunt Rostyd	Haddok
Wodecokke Roste	Freysse hake
Pertryche Roste	Solys y-sode
Plouer Roste	Gurnyd broylid with
	a syryppe
Snytys Roste	Brem de Mere
Grete byrdes Rosted	Roche
Larkys Rostyd	Perche
Vennysoun de Ro Rostyd	Menus fryid
Yrchouns	Yrchouns
	Elys y-rostyd
Vn leche	Leche lumbard
Payn puffe	Grete Crabbys
Colde bakemete	A cold bakemete[81]

Notes and References

1. Ian Kershaw, *Bolton Priory: The Economy of a Northern Monastery 1286–1325* (Oxford, 1973). See also the same author's *Bolton Priory Rentals and Ministers' Accounts 1473–1539* (Yorkshire Archaeological Society, Record Series 132, 1970 for 1969).

2. J. C. Dickinson, *The Origins of the Austin Canons and their Introduction into England* (London, 1950).
3. G. R. Price (ed.) and Stephen J. Whittle (transcriber), *The Court Rolls of Yeadon 1361–1476* (Draughton, 1984), pp. 227–47; William Brown (ed.), 'Description of the Buildings of Twelve Small Yorkshire Priories at the Reformation', *Yorkshire Archaeological and Topographical Journal* 9 (1886), pp. 321–5; H. C. Bell, 'Esholt Priory', *Yorkshire Archaeological Journal* 33 (1938), pp. 4–33.
4. John H. Tillotson, *Marrick Priory: A Nunnery in Late Medieval Yorkshire* (Borthwick Papers, 75 1989); T. S., 'Ground Plan and Charters of St. Andrew's Priory in the Parish of Marigg, North Riding, Co. Ebor', *Collectanea Topographica & Genealogica* 5 (1838), pp. 100–24 and 221–59. A copy of a plan of Marrick Priory is opposite p. 100. It is undated in this book, but if related to the other plan included was possibly made *c.*1592, when the Priory buildings were sold for the third time. T. M. Fallows suggested that the plan was taken at the time of the Dissolution: see William Page (ed.), *The Victoria County History of the County of York* 3 (1913, reprinted 1974), p. 117 n. 7.
5. John H. Tillotson, *Monastery and Society in the Late Middle Ages: Selected Account Rolls from Selby Abbey, Yorkshire, 1398–1537* (Woodbridge, Suffolk, 1988).
6. Ibid., p. 152.
7. David E. Owen, *Kirkstall Abbey* (Leeds, 1955), pp. 17–18. For further information on the Cistercians, see Tillotson (1988), pp. 6–7; and Louis J. Lekai, *The Cistercians: Ideals and Reality* (Kent State University Press, 1977).
8. George Zarnecki, 'The Monastic World: The Contribution of the Orders', *The Flowering of the Middle Ages*, ed. Joan Evans (London, 1966), p. 75.
9. Owen, p. 21.
10. Anthony Quiney, *The Traditional Buildings of England* (London, 1990), p. 155.
11. Kershaw (1973), pp. 14–17.
12. Tillotson (1988), pp. 16 and 18; Kershaw (1973), pp. 180–1.
13. Tillotson (1989), pp. 11 and 34–5; Tillotson (1988), pp. 158, 188–9, and 193; Kershaw (1973), pp. 147–8.
14. Tillotson (1988), pp. 9–12.
15. This has been established 'by the best authorities' as 0.5 l, said Lekai (p. 370). This is a little less than a modern English pint (20 fl. oz.), but more than the American pint equivalent to the older English wine pint (16 fl. oz.).
16. Kershaw (1973), pp. 132–3, 138, and 157–8.
17. Tillotson (1988), pp. 18 and 129–30; Tillotson (1989), p. 15.
18. Dickinson, p. 175.
19. Lekai, pp. 364–5.
20. Justin McCann (translator), *The Rule of St Benedict*, 2nd impression (London, 1978), p. 47. Note also *Three Middle-English Versions of the Rule of St Benet*, ed. Ernst A. Koch (Early English Text Society, OS 120, 1902).

21. David Knowles, *The Monastic Order in England* (Cambridge, 1949), pp. 456–7; Bridget Ann Henisch, *Fast and Feast*, pbk edn (Pennsylvania State University Press, 1985), pp. 20 and 32.
22. McCann, pp. 45–7. For *hemina*, see n. 15 above.
23. Knowles, pp. 462 and 464–5.
24. Owen, pp. 17–20.
25. This translates the Latin *emina* or *hemina*, which the footnote describes as 'a measure of liquid'. See note 15 above.
26. Walter Daniel, *The Life of Ailred of Rievaulx*, trans. F. M. Powick (London, 1950), pp. 10 and 11.
27. *The Register of William Wickwane, Lord Archbishop of York 1279–1285*, ed. William Brown (Surtees Society 114, 1907), pp. 132–3; Kershaw (1973), p. 9.
28. McCann, p. 55.
29. Dickinson, p. 181.
30. Harold Brakspear, *Waverley Abbey* (London, 1905), p. 90.
31. Knowles, pp. 458 and 462.
32. Chapter 53 of the Rule; McCann, pp. 57–9.
33. Knowles, pp. 457–9 and 461; Tillotson (1988), pp. 9 and 199; Henisch, p. 46; Lekai, pp. 375–6.
34. Dickinson, pp. 181–3.
35. Kershaw (1973), pp. 150–1; Tillotson (1988), pp. 461–2; Henisch, pp. 29–30.
36. Kershaw (1973), pp. 155–6, referring to Kingswood Abbey in Gloucestershire.
37. Brakspear, p. 69; Lekai, pp. 370–1.
38. Chapter 56 of the Rule; McCann, p. 61.
39. Tillotson (1989), p. 33; Tillotson (1988), p. 221.
40. Henisch, p. 52; Lekai, pp. 368–9.
41. Knowles, p. 463.
42. Tillotson (1988), pp. 58–65.
43. Knowles, p. 463; Kershaw (1973), pp. 142 and 145; in the same period, 265 quarters of bran went to feed the Priory's dog pack.
44. Tillotson (1988), pp. 142–4 and 145; pp. 243–4; and p. 189.
45. Tillotson (1989), p. 35.
46. McCann, pp. 41–2; *Three Middle-English Versions*, pp. 25–6, 31–2, 90–1, and 131–2.
47. Kershaw (1970), pp. 19–20; Price and Whittle , p. 237; Brown (1886), p. 324; Tillotson (1988), pp. 77–8.
48. Tillotson (1988), pp. 166–8 and 175. 'Skoinours' is so transcribed (p. 166), a vernacular word in the original Latin accounts. Perhaps 'skomours' (skimmers) is intended.
49. Tillotson (1988), pp. 165–6; Tillotson (1989), pp. 32–3. It is interesting to note the women employed at Selby apart from Agnes Bernard. Recorded in the Bursars' account of 1398–9 are Alice Trim, laundress for the Abbot, and Ellen de Helagh who mended and stitched his napery. The Pittancer, who provided money for the monks' robes, paid a laundress in 1441–2. The Granger of 1404–05 paid women who stacked turves in the Turfhouse. The

Kitchener in 1416–17 paid eight women to wash and shear 120
sheep. The Refectorer bought linen from Juliana Raghton and
Alice Ughtreth in 1421–2, and paid a laundress. The Infirmarer
also paid a laundress in 1401–2; Tillotson (1988), pp. 57, 66, 111,
138, 167, 196, and 201. This suggests that the ideal of the Rule,
which had the monks washing the towels after their week serving
in the kitchen, had given way by the fifteenth century to the
practice of paying women to do all the laundry.

50. There is a portrait of Master Robert, cook to Abbot Thomas de la
Mare (1349–96) of St Albans, included in a book of benefactors to
St Albans in 1380, following the record of a donation of 3s 4d by
his wife. He is depicted holding a broad kitchen knife (Henisch,
pp. 72–3).

51. *Three Middle-English Versions*, p. 27; McCann, pp. 41–2;
Tillotson (1988), pp. 194–7.

52. Lekai, p. 370.

53. Price and Whittle, pp. 237–40; Tillotson (1989), pp. 31–2 and 34;
Tillotson (1988), pp. 141–4.

54. Price and Whittle, pp. 237–40; Tillotson (1989), pp. 34–5;
Kershaw (1973), p. 146; Tillotson (1988), pp. 72, 144, and 145–7.

55. Tillotson (1988), p. 220; Tillotson (1989), p. 34.

56. Lekai, p. 339.

57. Kershaw (1973), pp. 150–5; Tillotson (1988), pp. 121–2 and
179–87.

58. Tillotson (1988), pp. 168–9 and 189–91.

59. Price and Whittle, p. 237; Tillotson (1989), p. 31; Kershaw
(1973), pp. 155 and 158; Tillotson (1988), pp. 187–8, 191, and
168.

60. Tillotson (1988), pp. 71–2, 136, and 178–9; Tillotson (1989),
p. 35.

61. Tillotson (1989), pp. 16 and 32; Tillotson (1988), pp. 167 and
168.

62. Kershaw (1973), p. 151.

63. Price and Whittle, pp. 237–9; Tillotson (1989), pp. 16 and 31.

64. Tillotson (1988), pp. 65–6, 163–4, 167, 168, and 192–3.

65. Ibid., pp. 134, 135, 136, 138, 148, and 178.

66. Kershaw (1973), pp. 146–7; Tillotson (1989), p. 35.

67. Tillotson (1988), p. 72–3, 122–3, 219, 223, and 225.

68. Kershaw (1973), p. 148; Tillotson (1988), pp. 163 and 166–9.

69. Brown (1886), pp. 321–5. A suggested reconstruction of the
ground plan, by W. T. Booth, can be found preceding the article by
Bell, p. 4.

70. *Collectanea Topographica* 5 (1838), pp. 239–56. The plan is
attached opposite p. 100.

71. There is a reconstructed plan of Waverley in the end pocket of
Brakspear's book.

72. Owen, pp. 20–35 and 50–4. The main source for this section,
apart from Owen's book, which was produced before the major
excavations had been completed, is *Kirkstall Abbey Excavations*

41

(Thoresby Society Publications, 43, 1950–4; 48, 1955–9; and 51, 1960–4). Related to these reports is an article by M. L. Ryder, 'The Animal Remains found at Kirkstall', *Agricultural History Review* 7 (1959), pp. 1–5. A later consideration of the excavation results is by Stephen Moorhouse and Stuart Wrathmell, *Kirkstall Abbey Volume 1: The 1950–64 Excavations, a Reassessment* (Wakefield, 1987). Further information on the Guesthouse excavation is provided by Stuart Wrathmell, *Kirkstall Abbey: The Guest House*, 2nd edn (Wakefield, 1987). Kirkstall Abbey was presented to the City of Leeds in 1889, and is administered by Leeds City Museum. Among the Museum's publications are the following two items by P. C. D. Brears: a booklet, *Kirkstall Abbey, Leeds' Cistercian Monastery* (Leeds, n.d.); and a leaflet including a bird's-eye view of the modern ruins, *Kirkstall Abbey* (Leeds, 1990).

73. W. H. St John Hope and J. Bilson, *Architectural Description of Kirkstall Abbey* (Thoresby Society Publications, 16, 1907), pp. 46–9; Owen, pp. 89–90.

74. Other alterations had been made to the warming house to the east of the refectory which are not considered here. For the alteration to the refectory and kitchen, see in particular Owen, pp. 41–4, 75–6, and 92–3; *Kirkstall Abbey Excavations* 43, pp. xi, 6, 7, 37–8, 39, 56, and 73; *Kirkstall Abbey Excavations* 48, pp. xiv, 2, 5–7, 29–30, 32–4, 35, 41–3, 47, 49, 56–7, 58–60, 62, 67–8, 70, 75, and 86; Moorhouse and Wrathmell, pp. 19–22, 24–5, 30, 36–9, 46, 49, and 152.

75. The original excavation report contains the suggestion that this may have been a slaughter house, as no other suitable site has been identified: *Kirkstall Abbey Excavation* 48, p. 62; but in retrospect a scullery seems the better solution.

76. With the monastic granges eventually rented out rather than worked directly by the monasteries, there was no need for the lay brothers; or alternatively, the fall in their numbers for other reasons may have prompted the lease of distant property. For a discussion on the lay brothers, see Lekai, pp. 334–44.

77. No remains of these hearths are now visible after excavation, and the floor area has been grassed over.

78. Compare Selby Abbey in 1416–17, when 383 sheep and 100 beef animals were consumed.

79. Quiney, pp. 191–2.

80. Moorhouse and Wrathmell, p. 56; Lekai, p. 318. Fish bones do not survive as easily as larger animal bones, and many that do are lost in excavation because they are so small. See A. Wheeler and A. Jones, *Fishes* (Cambridge Manual for Archaeology Series, 1989).

81. *Two Fifteenth-Century Cookery-Books*, ed. T. Austin (Early English Text Society, OS 91, 1888), pp. 61–2.

3.

Keeping Hospitality and Board Wages: Servants' Feeding Arrangements from the Middle Ages to the Nineteenth Century

C. ANNE WILSON

As Sir Gawain rode into north-western England on his way to the green chapel, where he was pledged to meet the green knight, he saw a castle on the horizon set in a park with a strong paling round it. At once he gave thanks to Jesus and St Julian, adding, 'Now *bone hostel* I beseech you grant.'[1] Underlying the words *bone hostel*, which can be modernised as 'good lodging' or 'good hospitality', is the very wide-ranging concept of hospitality already in operation among the nobility and the gentry families of the later Middle Ages.[2] The households of these families were so organised that they were ready to supply meals and lodging not only for kinsfolk and invited guests but also for passing travellers (usually travellers who belonged to a similar social sphere to that of the host family); and meals at least were available for daily visitors such as workpeople, and those who came on estate business. All this was made possible by a very large network of servants.

Moreover, the guests themselves arrived with servants of their own – grooms for the horses, their personal or body servants, and a few extra servants as an escort, who wore the livery of the guest and rode on his well-kept horses, thereby emphasising his important status to passers-by as well as to the host. We have a glimpse of such a visitation in a letter of Richard Cely written to his brother from his parents' home in Essex in 1479: 'and here has been Coldale

43

and his wife and divers of my lord's men, and dined with our father and were merry'.[3]

The household servants were responsible for purchasing and preparing the food and serving the meals, as well as for the other duties that had to be performed to keep the household and its estate running smoothly. Who were these servants? Many of them were the sons of gentlemen of similar rank to the head of the household where they served, who would later inherit estates of their own; or they were younger sons hoping to make useful contacts during their service.[4] The household still reflected its military origin, and the servants of peacetime would follow their lord into battle, wearing his badge and colours should the need ever arise. Within the castle or great house an upper servant often had a room of his own, and one or more servants attached to him to look after *his* needs (though they were forbidden to carry out his duties for him).

There were very few women in the household. The lord's wife had one or two ladies of similar rank (either young, unmarried gentlewomen or wives of members of the household) as companions, and one or two ladies of lower rank to act as chamberers. If the lord frequently left his main abode to visit his other castles, taking with him his riding household but leaving behind his lady, then she might have a household of her own, smaller than his but with similar posts of steward and other upper servants, all of them men. The only other woman to have a position in the household was the laundress; she usually lived outside and came in to perform her duties. The rest of the housework was carried out by men. It should be recalled that there was very much less of it to be done in the Middle Ages than in any later period, as there were fewer furnishings to be cared for, and some of them, such as bedding and wall-hangings, were removed and stored temporarily during that part of the day when they were not needed. Young boys did some of the other necessary tasks. High-born boys were henchmen, and their duties were mainly ceremonial; but some of the pages were of humbler origins, and they did various kitchen or kitchen-related jobs, such as turning the spit and dusting nightly in the pantry.[5]

There could be one or two hundred (or even more) servants in a large household. Even the smallest manorial households usually had at least twenty. Most of the servants were expected to eat together in the Great Hall, seated at tables with other servants of their own rank, including visiting servants of appropriate rank when any were present. The exceptions were the porter, who ate in his lodge at the gate, and the servants concerned with the preparation and serving of the meal. Thus, in a great household the yeoman baker would eat in his bakehouse if he was still at work baking when dinner was served; the master cook and his assistants would eat in the kitchen after the final course had been served in the hall; and the ushers, sewar, and butler, who organised the seating arrangements and the meal service, also had their own meal separately, usually eating after their fellow servants.[6]

In the household of George, Duke of Clarence, according to the ordinances of 1469, it was the almoner and his yeoman and grooms who were responsible for serving the tables in the main body of the hall where the servants sat, making sure that 'every two persons be served out of the pantry with a cheat loaf; eight persons with a gallon of ale out of the buttery . . . and a mess of meat sufficiently filled from the kitchen for four persons'.[7] Just how much meat or fish was contained in a mess is problematical. Christopher Dyer has suggested 'calculating a typical mess as about 2 lbs of bread, between 6 and 8 pints of ale, and 3 or 4 lb of meat or fish'.[8] The amount of ale, at least, is higher than that prescribed for the Duke of Clarence's household.

In the rather austere household of the Princess Cecil, mother of King Edward IV, the service at dinner on Sunday, Tuesday, and Thursday was of 'boiled beef and mutton (probably boiled in pottage with oatmeal and herbs) and one roast; at supper, lechyd (sliced) beef and mutton roast . . .

upon fasting days, salt fish and two dishes of fresh fish; if there come a principal feast, it is served like unto the feast honourably'.[9] On feast days a much greater variety of fleshmeat was eaten, including boar, venison, capons, pigeons, and wild birds of many kinds. Some of the scarce or highly valued items were confined to the high table, but the servants in the main body of the hall received a share of many of the special dishes.

Although one mess of meat supplied four men among the lesser servants, it might be assigned to three, two, or even a single person among the top office-holders in a great household. These important people were thus given the option of eating more than their lowlier fellows, or at least selecting the choicest parts of the mess they received. The mess itself could consist of several dishes. Queen Elizabeth I's treasurer and her comptroller each had '10 dishes of meat to his first mess and 6 dishes to his second, every meal'. The yeoman of the counting-house, on the other hand, received 'three dishes of meat every meal, for him and his fellow the groom'.[10]

Similar variation is found in the amount of the liveries of bread and ale or beer issued daily to servants; high-ranking servants received wine in addition. The liveries were taken away to the servant's workplace, or chamber of office if he held a high office, and they were thus available if he felt the need for refreshment between meals or in the late evening. When hospitality was being kept at the Yorkshire castles of the fifth Earl of Northumberland, his chamberlain, steward, treasurer, and controller each received a livery of a manchet (small loaf of finest wheat flour), half a loaf of household bread, a pottle (2 quarts) of beer, and a quart of wine. The gentlemen ushers, by contrast, were given no more than a quarter of a loaf of household bread and a quart of beer; while the yeomen waiters and the yeomen and grooms of the household who assisted the gentlemen officers, and who shared a single chamber, also shared the livery granted to that chamber of a loaf of household bread and a pottle of beer.[11] The size of the liveries given to the most senior officials meant that they could, without hesitation, have offered a drink to a visitor, even if they were visited in their own chambers by several different people in the course of a day.

By the fifteenth century the lord and his lady and their personal guests were dining regularly in the Great Chamber, and no longer in the Great Hall with the rest of the household, except on special feast days. The steward now presided over the table on the dais in the hall, where he entertained those guests not grand enough to be invited to the meal in the chamber. The principal ushers, yeomen of the chamber, sewars, cupbearers, and carvers carried the dishes of a fine dinner from the kitchen to the chamber, while their grooms and pages served out simpler fare to the household servants and visiting tenants and workmen in the hall. It was the prerogative of the staff who served at the lord's table to receive the reversion, or remains, of the lavish spread after the main meal was over. This system was probably based on ancient custom, but appears in the written household regulations only when they are exceptionally detailed. In the *Northumberland Household Book*, compiled for the fifth Earl of Northumberland in 1512, the list of 'the persons to await at meals in my Lord's chamber and to have the reversion' numbers twelve men, including the almoner, the carver, the sewar, two cupbearers, a gentleman waiter, four yeomen, a henchman for various waiting duties, and finally the groom of the chamber who kept the door. A further group of ten servants, including yeomen, grooms, and clerks, was appointed to 'sit in the hall at dinner in my Lord's dinner-time and to await at after dinner', that is, they were the servants who would wait on those men who had already waited at the Lord's table when they sat at the second or after dinner and consumed the reversion.[12]

Still more complicated were the arrangements at the Scottish court, after King James VI married Anne of Denmark in 1590. The king and queen ate at separate tables, probably in separate chambers, and their reversions, described as their 'rests', went to separate groups of attendants – the king's to the 'gentlemen servandis table' and the queen's to the first master householder's table of ten men. These in their turn were waited on by the queen's four pages and five other people, who then received their reversion or 'rests'.[13] Some household books suggest that the final remains of the food from the lord's table went back to the kitchen for consumption by the cook's assistants. But Queen Henrietta Maria's regulations of 1627 first instruct the usher 'when the meat is taken from the table to call the pages to carry it to the waiters' chamber, giving them charge not to suffer it to be diminished, but to be kept for the waiters'; and subsequently require 'that one of the pages stay in the chamber after the waiters have dined or supped, to see the reversion duly served on the tables for the servants that are there allowed, and to suffer no other to stay in the chamber'.[14] Those servants, probably the personal servants of the waiters, may have tasted some fine dishes of food, but only at third hand, when they had been well picked over and were presumably quite cold. The reversion system did, however, have the advantage of preventing wastage of the lavish quantities of food served at the principal table, and it was incorporated into calculations for expenditure of food. Those who received reversions received nothing else for their main meals except bread and ale (or bread and wine for the men holding the highest offices).

Periodically, the lord and his lady and his riding household (a smaller group of servants than the complete household) departed from one residence to visit another castle or house belonging to him, or else to stay for a time in the household of one of his kinsmen or friends. Then hospitality was no longer kept in the house they left behind. Most of the remaining servants were put on board wages. These were, of course, graded according to rank, and for the lowest paid would over a year have totalled far more than their annual salary. Queen Elizabeth I's clerk of the kitchen received

£44 6s 8d a year, and 20d. a day board wages; while the
'children' or young boys who were on the staff of the
serjeant of the scullery and whose job was 'to make clean
[the] dishes' and to wait on the kitchen workers at their
mealtimes, received £2 a year each and 6d a day for board
wages.[15] The lower servants who stayed on in the house in a
caretaking capacity would have pooled their board wages,
but even so could only afford a cheaper and duller diet than
they enjoyed when the full household was present; no more
fresh beef, but basic bread and ale, with some bacon and
perhaps mutton from a 'stock' animal, that is, one culled
from the lord's flock pastured nearby.[16]

For a rare glimpse of a household with only one servant
we can turn to the account book of the two priests of
Munden's Chantry at Bridport.[17] The income for their
small household came partly from the endowments left by
John Munden, and partly from the rents of the tenants of
properties owned by the Chantry, and they purchased all
their food and drink apart from some garden produce and
the occasional food gift. They regularly enjoyed beef,
mutton, and pork on fleshdays, and a variety of fresh and
salt fish on fishdays. Their high consumption of oatmeal
suggests that pottages were frequently on their menu. The
priests sometimes had guests for dinner, and quite often
they shared their meals with workpeople such as carpenters,
thatchers, and masons, each with his own 'servant' or mate
(the men may have been carrying out repairs on the
Chantry's tenements).

Small as the house may have been, its hall contained two
long tables and one little one. This would have allowed for
the typical medieval division of a high table, where the
priests sat, together with their own guests when any were
present, and a separate long table for the workpeople; while
the little table could have been utilised as a cupboard for the
'2 great basins with two ewers' for handwashing before and
after meals, and for cups for the ale, and occasionally wine
for the upper table, which always accompanied the food.[18]

The single servant, having acted as waiter at both long tables, presumably had to feed upon the reversion afterwards in the kitchen where he had prepared the meal in the first place. Perhaps this was one reason for the remarkably high turnover in holders of the post. No fewer than ten different men acted as servant to the priests in the seven years between 1453 and 1460.

A great many servants worked for humbler households, such as those of small-scale tenant farmers and peasant landowners. They were often young people who 'lived with their employers and who received much of their pay in the form of their keep . . . They were regarded as part of the family, and indeed often were related to their employers.'[19] When such families worked at harvest time for manorial lords, the servants went with them, and shared in the usually substantial food allowances given to workers at harvest time. Surviving records indicate that in the thirteenth century harvest workers received bread of local grain, often maslin (wheat mixed with rye) or barley, accompanied by cheese, bacon, or saltfish; but by the fifteenth century wheat bread was more usual, at least in lowland Britain, with beef, mutton, or fresh fish supplying the protein element. These changes in the direction of the diet chosen in more wealthy households possibly reflected similar changes in the ordinary daily diet of village folk at other times of year, as Dyer has suggested.[20] But in the absence of more direct evidence it is probably safer to assume that cheese and bacon still played a big part in their everyday meals and in those of their servants. Nevertheless, wheat bread was becoming more common, especially in towns, where the servants of wealthy merchants would have been able to enjoy it regularly, and even the servants of small-scale traders and artisans must have eaten it from time to time.

Servants in the humbler households in both town and country were often women. Girls and women from poor families who needed to take paid employment chose domestic service when such work was available, even though they earned less than a man doing the same job, because they received their keep as well as a small wage. This arrangement may often have given them a higher standard of living than they could have hoped for at home. Under the Tudors, for reasons partly economic and partly political, women began to be employed as servants in gentry households and even, to a limited extent, in the households of the nobility.

The great medieval household reached its peak, in terms of the number of servants employed, about the mid-fifteenth century. At that time the most important noble families kept 300 or 400 men, and even lesser gentry families might have had fifty or sixty, the majority of them concerned with servicing their fellow servants rather than with the direct needs of the family at the head. The cost had to be met from the rents and produce of the family's estates, and eventually these could no longer support the burden. Furthermore, under the Tudors the court became the focal point, and the place where important contacts were made. A member of the nobility or gentry could take only a few servants with him when he visited the court; the rest remained behind, often in a fine new country house he had recently built. But in the divided household, which was also reduced in size, the upper servants in the country residence no longer had a political role to play in acting as messengers to, and negotiators with, other great households; and members of the aristocracy and gentry were less eager to let their sons take on a servant's role in a household no longer a centre of regional influence. Increasingly the servants engaged came of yeoman stock or were women, who were cheaper to employ than men.

Often the women were wives of household employees. The beginning of this new trend can be seen in the household accounts of the Lestranges, a gentry family living at Hunstanton. In 1519 a payment of 8*d* was made to the neatherd's wife 'for 5 weeks helping the cook in the kitchen'. By the following year there is a new kitchen boy to help the cook, and several payments are made for items of clothing for him.[21] But eventually women were to find more than temporary employment in the kitchens of great houses. Shakespeare's Mistress Quickly, servant to Dr Caius in *The Merry Wives of Windsor* is perhaps the first recorded housekeeper, for she says: 'I keep his house; and I wash, wring, brew, bake, scour, dress meat and drink, make the beds and do all myself'.[22]

For a time the servants in the great houses continued to eat in the Great Hall, where the high table had become known as the steward's table. There the steward sat with the other upper servants, and entertained visitors of appropriate rank. The *Northumberland Household Book* of 1512 shows that the steward's table in the Percy family's Yorkshire castles received a more varied diet than the other tables in the hall where the rest of the servants sat. At the steward's table chickens, hens, and pigeons were sometimes served, and conies and capons too when guests were present;[23] the lower servants would have been limited to beef and mutton except on very special occasions. An account by a Venetian visitor who came to England about 1500 includes the comment: '. . . the English, being great epicures and very avaricious by nature, indulge in the most delicate fare themselves, and give their household the coarsest bread and beer and cold meat baked on Sunday for the week, which, however, they allow them in great abundance'.[24]

Eating arrangements for servants were beginning to change even before the end of the sixteenth century. The new country houses were constructed with a smaller entrance hall; although some of the servants could still eat there, sitting at their temporary trestle tables which were taken down and removed when the meal was over, others were expected to dine in their work-places, such as the kitchen or the laundry. The Berkeley household accounts for the 1580s illustrate this trend, with messes being sent to various different locations for the servants.[25]

For a time the Great Chamber continued to be the eating place for the family, but it was beginning to be superseded by a new dining parlour or dining room, at least for less formal meals. In houses where the family continued to eat in the Great Chamber, the parlour might be allotted to the upper servants, who thus began to eat not only apart from the other servants but also in superior accommodation. The final change for the lower servants was the institution of the servants' hall as a separate room from the entrance hall, and built on the storey below it, next to the kitchen and other food offices, and at garden level. This innovation did not come about until the second half of the seventeenth century.[26] By that time the family dining room and saloon were usually arranged to open off the entrance hall; and the servants carried the dishes for the family's meals up a purpose-built staircase leading from the kitchen level, and consumed their own meals in the servants' hall.

The arrangements for servants in small houses were, of course, simpler. Farm servants, who often lodged in the farmhouse, ate in the kitchen with the farmer and his family, but they sat at a separate table further from the fire. Henry Best's farm account book, compiled at Elmswell in the East Riding of Yorkshire in 1641, describes the different types of grain sent from his farm to the mill to be ground for household use, and it is clear that distinctions in quality between the food for the family and the food for the servants were maintained on the farm just as they were in the houses of the nobility. 'We send for our own pies a bushel of the best wheat', he wrote. 'We send for the folk's puddings a bushel of barley . . . in harvest time they have wheat puddings. The folk's pie crusts are made of maslin, as our bread is . . . In many places they grind the after-loggings of wheat for their servants' pies.'[27] It is also clear that meat was eaten more sparingly on the farm than at the great house, being eked out by the flour and lard of the pie crusts and the flour and suet of the puddings.

During the seventeenth century the concept of 'keeping

hospitality' was losing its medieval connotation of a widespread generosity in entertaining all comers, with the further underlying objective of demonstrating to the guests the power, influence, and wealth of the host. As time went on, hospitality grew to be more of a reciprocal activity conducted between friends and with kinsfolk. When it took place in great houses the visitors might still arrive with a large supporting cast of servants, but they were now prepared to make some recompense for the expense that such an influx brought to the household. The records of the Bedford family at Woburn Abbey from 1667 onwards show that when the married children came back for lengthy visits they paid their way. An entry for 1671 begins: 'Received of Mr William Russell for the diet and entertainment of himself, his lady and retinue from Lady Day, 1670, to the 9th of June then next following at £8 the week – £88.' A further payment to cover the next three months was reduced by £1 10s a week for six weeks when three of their servants were absent, thus indicating that the cost of each servant's board and lodging was reckoned at 10s a week.[28] Servants who were not staying in a great house but merely calling there to deliver a gift or message could no longer, as in medieval times, expect to join the household at dinner. They penetrated no further than the buttery bar (near the entrance, and moved to garden entrance level when the kitchen was established at that level), where they were given bread and cheese along with a drink of beer before they went on their way.

Board wages, however, were still as much a part of life in the larger household as they had been in the Middle Ages. Then the lord and his lady departed with their riding household to stay in another of their castles, or to become the guests of another powerful lord. In the later seventeenth and eighteenth centuries the family was more likely to set off for Bath to spend a few weeks taking the waters, or else to make an extended visit to the home of a relative. But in either case the servants who remained at home were put onto board wages.

Variations in the rates of board wages were maintained, as they had been since medieval times. In Queen Elizabeth I's household the clerk of the kitchen's board wage was over three times the amount paid to a yeoman of the great bakehouse or to a 'child' in the scullery.[29] In later centuries the differential both in salaries and board wages narrowed somewhat, especially in middling or smaller sized households, but upper servants continued to receive more than lower servants; and women servants, who were increasingly employed in gentry households, received less than men servants. Webster's *Encyclopaedia of Domestic Economy* of 1844 states that 'board wages for men vary according to the circumstances of the family paying them, from twelve to fourteen shillings per week; for women, from eight shillings to twelve per week'.

Webster goes on to define the three modes of operation of board wages:

> Servants living on board wages usually club together
> and appoint the cook of the family to be their caterer;
> or, in some cases, the cook contracts with the rest to
> provide them at so much per head their dinners and
> suppers. A third arrangement is sometimes adopted.
> Food generally is provided for the establishment, but
> money is allowed each servant to provide for himself
> beer, sugar and tea . . . Of these modes the principals
> of families adopt that which to each family
> respectively appears to be most convenient or
> economical. Servants have no choice in the matter,
> farther than that of declining to serve in families
> where arrangements of this nature appear to them
> objectionable, or not conducted in a manner likely to
> promote their daily comfort.[30]

The first two arrangements which made the cook responsible for catering as well as for cooking would have been well suited to large estates, where the cook could bargain for estate produce with the steward or bailiff, for bacon, salt fish, and other foods 'in store' with the clerk of the kitchen, and for ale or beer with the butler. It is likely that both these methods of living on board wages were traditional and had continued since medieval times. The third arrangement suited the families in lesser country houses, where the consumption of meat, eggs, milk, butter, cheese, and vegetables from the estate could follow the usual pattern but on a reduced scale when the servants were left on their own. Dorothy Yorke at Erddig in Denbighshire wrote to her son Philip in November 1765 about her negotiations over the servants' board wages (finally fixed at 4*s* a week for the men and 3*s* for the maids), and added: 'They are to find nothing for themselves but ale, sugar and bread, and they have some small stock to begin with. This will prevent strangers soaking there whilst we are gone, as too many have got on that footing at Erddig.'[31]

Eventually some families began to give board wages to their servants on a full-time basis in the belief that to do so would be an economy and would also save trouble. But this system proved to have disadvantages. Mrs W. Parkes, in the second edition of *Domestic Duties* (1825), wrote that servants

> cannot work well, unless they have food enough, and this with me is a sufficient argument against board wages, which seldom supply them with more than a very moderate portion of food, besides increasing the inducements to obtain by dishonest means an additional allowance of the essentials of life.[32]

Webster's *Encyclopaedia of Domestic Economy* contains a similar criticism of permanent board wages as 'a mode full of temptation to petty thieving in servants scarcely to be resisted, and hence its evils are greater than its advantages'.[33]

So in many, and perhaps most, households the servants' food was provided for them when the family was in residence, and their wages were adjusted accordingly. Their mealtime arrangements underwent some changes. In medieval times the placement of the servants within the Great Hall had been organised on a hierarchical basis: every servant (apart from the cooks and the various ushers and waiters) sat at a table 'with persons of like service', whether he was knight, esquire, yeoman, groom, or page.[34] During the sixteenth and seventeenth centuries, when the Great Hall was reduced in size and importance, the servants were divided at mealtimes, with some eating in or near their principal place of work. But by the end of the seventeenth century a new hierarchical system was emerging. In the greatest houses the house-steward had his own room; in smaller country houses the housekeeper had taken over the steward's role of responsibility for the smooth running of the household, and she likewise had her own housekeeper's room. The upper servants gathered in the steward's or housekeeper's room to eat their breakfasts and suppers, and also an afternoon tea meal which was eventually instituted to fill the gap between dinner and supper. The other servants took their meals in the servants' hall. Only for dinner did the upper servants join the lower servants in their hall.

Dinner was the main meal in the servants' day, always consumed at the end of their morning's work, even when the fashionable dining hour for their employers had moved forward, first to the late afternoon and then to the early evening. Immediately after the main meat course at dinner the upper servants rose and followed the steward or housekeeper out of the hall and back to his or her room, where they enjoyed a second course based on the leftovers from the delicacies that had been served on the family's table upstairs. Occasionally, in the case of a big London household, the delicacies came direct to the steward's table, or second table as it was often called, having been obtained

5.
Upper servants at
the second table,
from *A Treatise on
the Use and Abuse
of the Second
Table* (London,
c.1750).

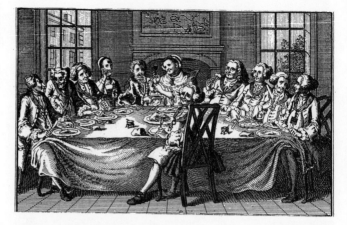

by the steward with the connivance of the butcher, the fishmonger, or other food traders, on the family's account.[35] Retailers were keen to supply provisions to the big households on a regular basis, and encouraged stewards and housekeepers to patronise them by offering perks in the form of food or money. This could happen even in a smallish country household. The Yorke family at Erddig were very surprised when the will of their housekeeper, Mary Webster, who died in 1875, revealed savings of £1,300.[36] This sum, much more than she could have earned in her thirty years' service, may well have been made up in part from back-handers from the shopkeepers of Wrexham.

The select group of upper servants who sat at the second table in a large eighteenth-century household might include the house-steward, the clerk of the kitchen, the clerk of the stables, the butler, the groom of the chambers, the French valet, and the French cook. The land-steward and the head gardener sat with them, unless they chose to eat at home in their own houses. The housekeeper and the lady's personal maid were the only female servants there.[37] In a smaller establishment the group of upper servants comprised the housekeeper (replacing the steward), the lady's maid, the cook (who might also be female), the valet, the butler, and the land-steward or bailiff, if he ate at the second table rather than at home.

The footmen, coachman, and grooms, and the house-maids, kitchenmaids, nurserymaids, and laundrymaids made up the community of lower servants who ate in the servants' hall. They too could look forward to receiving leftovers from the upstairs meals as an addition to their everyday food, once the second table had been satisfied. Not surprisingly, there were many stories of footmen quickly removing the plates of the family's guests, so they should have no chance of a second helping from an especially delectable dish: 'away flies the plate, and is immediately replaced by a clean one, a plain hint for him to choose something else'.[38]

The delicious dishes from upstairs supplemented the servants' usual diet which is recorded in some household accounts. Meat was very important, and in wealthy households it was offered to them on a prodigal scale. In the early eighteenth century the servants of the Duke of Chandos at Canons, near Edgware, were each allowed an average of 21 oz. of beef on Tuesdays, Thursdays, and Sundays; 21 oz. of mutton on Mondays and Fridays; and 14 oz. of pork on Wednesdays and Saturdays.[39] In lesser households, too, even the lower servants were supplied abundantly with fleshmeat and received bread and ale to accompany it. But at some houses such servants were said to be 'debarred of a vegetable support necessary to dilute the acrimonious particles of flesh. I mean greens, potatoes and roots of all kinds.'[40] The upper servants presumably acquired their vegetable support from among the side dishes left over from the family's meals.

In smaller households the servants' dinner was more likely to come from a meat animal which was also supplying the family's needs on that day. Reminders for the cook at Erddig Hall have survived which show that on Tuesday, 13 October 1730, the dinner ordered for Mr Meller (then owner of the Hall) and his guests was: 'A fry'd sole, stewed apples, sallet, goose roasted, ribs of beef roasted', with 'Boil'd beef for ye Hall', that is, the servants' hall. For dinner on a Wednesday in September 1732, Mr Meller had: 'Knuckle of veal & bacon, loin of mutton roasted, pudding', with 'Leg of mutton boiled for ye Hall'.[41]

A frugal Scottish diet for servants was recorded by Lady Grisell Baillie in her *Household Book* in 1752, for her 'common servants' at Mellerstain, a few miles from Kelso.

> Sunday they have boiled beef and broth made in the great pot, and always the broth made to serve two days. Monday broth made on Sunday and a herring. Tuesday broth and beef. Wednesday broth and 2 eggs each. Thursday broth and beef. Friday broth and herring. Saturday broth without meat, and cheese, or a pudding or blood puddings, or a haggis, or what is most convenient. In the big pot for the 2 days broth is allowed 2 pound of barley or groats, or half and half.

The beef in the broth for Lady Grisell's 'common servants' was salt beef, and the quantity allowed was 1 lb per head. 'No allowance in that for the second table', she wrote, 'they getting what comes from the first table'. Elsewhere she gave directions to the butler that he should 'let not the dirty china [from the dining room] go into the kitchen till the cook be ready to clean it and empty the meat of them into pewter dishes before it goes to the second table'.[42]

In England in the nineteenth century the accent was still upon a substantial daily allowance of meat for servants. The author of the *Housekeeper's Oracle* wrote in 1829: 'There is much more meat, &c. ate in the kitchen than there is in the parlour.'[43] The kitchen was, of course, the eating place for servants in houses too small to have a separate servants' hall. Shortly before, Mrs Parkes had summed up the servants' diet thus:

Their meals should be at regular and early hours;
their food plain, substantial and good. Butcher's meat
once a day is the general allowance for servants in the
establishments of those of moderate fortunes, with
cheese for supper. The cook, however, should be
desired to reserve such pieces of cold meat as would
not be sent into the dining-room, for the supper of
the men-servants, which, now and then, will prevent
the cutting up of a large piece of cheese, and be also a
more wholesome and nutritious meal.[44]

No specific quantities are suggested, but it was as well for a
master and mistress to have a reputation for generosity in
the matter of the meat supply if they wished to attract and
keep good domestic staff. As for the great house, Castle Hill
in Devon, home of the Earls Fortescue, was not untypical:
the daily allowance of food for servants there in the 1850s
included 1½ lb of meat for each one, together with 1 lb of
flour, a quart of ale, and a pint of small beer.[45]

Ale and beer had been the traditional drinks for servants
since the Middle Ages, and for manservants this tradition
was continued right to the end of the nineteenth century.
At that date there were still many households where beer
was the only drink available to them, not only with dinner
and supper but also at breakfast time.[46] Economy was an
underlying cause: tea and sugar remained expensive until
well into the nineteenth century, whereas beer was brewed
at home in the larger establishments where there were
many servants, thus requiring outlay only on the basic
barley and hops. Beer was often available on a generous
scale, for the servants' physical work created large thirsts;
but this led in turn to problems of alcoholism. At Cannon
Hall a few miles from Barnsley, home of the Spencer-
Stanhopes, for instance, in the late eighteenth century not
only was beer allowed to the servants in unlimited quantities
at mealtimes but water-jugs full of beer were also placed in
the manservants' bedrooms for their refreshment at other

times – clearly a legacy of the medieval practice of granting each servant a livery of ale to take away to his work-place or room to quench his thirst between meals. At Cannon Hall, too, a special superior brew was allowed to the second table, and as the upper servants passed from the servants' hall to the housekeeper's room after the main course of dinner, 'the custom was for them to "sink their beer", viz. throw the inferior beverage out of the glasses which they carried with them into the sink, in order to claim the better drink which awaited them'.[47]

Safe water was not available as an alternative to beer until quite late in the nineteenth century. But in the north of England and Scotland milk was sometimes given to servants in households where cows were kept on the estate, and a surplus of milk reached the dairy at certain seasons. Lady Grisell Baillie offered her servants for breakfast and supper 'a mutchkin [12 fl. oz.] of beer, or milk whenever there is any'.[48] During the nineteenth century the amount of beer issued to servants in England became more regulated; in mid-century it was usually set at 1 pint at each meal for men and half a pint for women.[49]

Tea-drinking became popular during the early years of the eighteenth century, very much as a women's activity and it was women servants who helped to popularise it. The housekeeper and the waiting-woman or lady's maid were keen to imitate the lady of the house and her friends in drinking tea, and the lower servants imitated the upper servants. In 1752 it was claimed that 'it is now usual with many female servants to insist on tea in their agreement, and to refuse serving where that is not allowed'.[50] Many mistresses of households preferred to pay a tea allowance in cash; typical sums are a wage of 6 guineas a year plus 1 guinea for tea paid to a housemaid in the 1770s, and a wage of £23 a year 'plus 2 guineas for tea' paid to the cook-housekeeper at Englefield House, Berkshire, in 1800.[51] These sums indicate that the upper servants could afford to buy tea of a higher quality than could the lower servants.

The third edition of *A New System of Practical Domestic Economy* (1823) stated that

> In most families, all the servants except those in the nursery find their own tea and sugar, for which an adequate consideration is made to them in their wages . . . In families in which tea is allowed to the female servants, one pound will serve seven or eight persons a week very well, which is about two ounces a week each.[52]

In 1861, when Mrs Beeton published *The Book of Household Management*, the tea allowance in cash was still being paid in some families, while others paid a lower wage but provided tea.[53] The cash allowance was still approximately £2 for upper female servants and £1 for lower ones, but now covered not only tea but sugar and beer as well, reflecting both the decrease in the price of tea since the early years of the century and the reduction in the number of houses where beer was now home-brewed.

Main meals for servants usually took place at fixed times. In the mid-nineteenth century these were commonly 8.00 a.m. for breakfast, 12.30 or 1.00 p.m. for dinner, and 8.00 p.m. for supper, with the servants summoned to each meal by 'the ringing of a great bell', according to Webster's *Encyclopaedia of Domestic Economy*.[54] But this regime was relaxed at times when the servants entertained their friends, or they themselves went out to be entertained.

A certain amount of unofficial hospitality was lavished by servants upon their friends and relatives when their master and mistress were away from home and unaware of what was going on. Beer or tea and bread were the refreshments most readily offered to visitors, whether casual or invited (hence Dorothy Yorke's desire to put her servants at Erddig on board wages for bread and ale during her absence in 1765). But in some households all sorts of foodstuffs were smuggled out to hangers-on by the servants even when the family was at home, if the master and mistress were lax and did not insist that proper accounts for food be kept and vetted regularly. Upper servants in some of the great houses managed to entertain their own friends upon superior fare at the second table, and even to give extravagant parties.[55]

There were, however, occasions when employers themselves were ready to make extra provision for the hospitality offered in the servants' hall. The coachmen and footmen who accompanied the family's own dinner guests were given supper there with the home servants, and whiled away the evening drinking beer with them. This led inevitably to cases of inebriation, and stories have come down of coachmen too drunk to drive their people home at the end of the evening;[56] in the eighteenth century their port-drinking masters were often in no better state themselves.

Rather different were the occasions when visiting workmen carrying out tasks for the estate were invited to a meal in the servants' hall. Dorothy Yorke wrote from Erddig to her son Philip in July 1769:

> all the slates of your mill was brought last Friday, 23 carters dined in your servants hall, near 50 men with carters, and I endeavoured to please them with plum pudden and beef sufficient with your strong beer and ale.[57]

Beef and plum pudding was a favourite combination for a celebratory meal for the home servants, too, on other country estates, especially during the Christmas season.[58]

Finally, it is pleasant to record that many employers were prepared from time to time to provide entertainment for their servants, either among themselves or with friends they invited from outside. In this it is possible to recognise a partial continuation of the old concept of 'keeping hospitality', as it had been understood in late medieval and Tudor times. Longleat is an example of a great house where servants were treated in this considerate fashion. Dances were held for the staff there every Tuesday and Thursday in the late nineteenth century, where the outdoor servants joined the indoor ones, and they all enjoyed a buffet supper prepared by the kitchen and stillroom workers.[59]

In smaller households it was not unusual for servants to be permitted to invite friends or relatives to come and drink tea with them in the servants' hall or the housekeeper's room; sometimes the visitors would stay for the evening, to talk or play cards and to share the servants' supper, and if there were a musician present with a fiddle or other instrument, the evening might end with an hour or two of dancing.[60] References to such happenings are found in the diaries and letters of their employers, and one of the most charming comes from the diary of Parson Woodforde. He was often generous in allowing the servants in his small household free time to spend with their friends who called at the house, or with friends outside. An entry in his diary in 1792 runs:

There was a frolic given to the servants at Weston House this afternoon, tea and supper, etc. Our servants were invited, Betty and Breton went about five in the afternoon and stayed until eleven at night. Our people said they were never at a better frolic.[61]

Notes and References

1. *Sir Gawain and the Green Knight*, ed. T. Silverstein (Chicago and London, 1974), 1. 776.
2. F. Heal, *Hospitality in Early Modern England* (Oxford, 1990), p. 23. This book is a major study of the concepts and practice of hospitality in late medieval and early modern England, both of which have undergone considerable change since.
3. *The Cely Letters*, ed. A. Hanham (Early English Text Society, OS 273, 1975), no. 55, 1. 20-1.
4. The servants often came from local gentry families, but were rarely related to the lord, cf. Lord Burghley's warning to his son, 'Be not served with kinsmen and friends, for they expect much and do little', *Household Papers of Henry Percy, 9th Earl of Northumberland*, ed. G. R. Botho (Camden 3rd ser. 93, 1962), p. xxiv.
5. K. Mertes, *The Noble English Household, 1250-1600* (Oxford,

C. ANNE WILSON

1988), p. 30, and *passim* for the arrangement of the household and the duties of the servants.

6. The yeomen and grooms who acted as waiters to their fellow-servants of similar rank received similar food in the hall, and were waited on by pages or 'children' of the scullery. The sewar, cupbearer, usher, and others carrying out waiting and serving duties for the lord's table in the hall or chamber received the reversion (discussed below).

7. *A Collection of Ordinances and Regulations for the Government of the Royal Household made in Divers Reigns* (London, 1790), p. 90.

8. C. Dyer, *Standards of Living in the Later Middle Ages* (Cambridge, 1989), p. 64.

9. *Collection of Ordinances and Regulations*, p. 38.

10. Ibid., pp. 281–2.

11. *The Regulations and Establishment of the Household of Henry Algernon Percy, the Fifth Earl of Northumberland . . . 1512* (London, 1827), pp. 97–8.

12. Ibid., pp. 300–2, 362–3.

13. A. Gibson and T. C. Smout, 'Food and Hierarchy in Scotland, 1550–1650', in L. Leneman (ed.), *Perspectives in Scottish Social History* (Aberdeen, 1988), pp. 34–5. The further remains passed to cooks, probably, and to other servants (ibid., table on p. 38).

14. *Collection of Ordinances and Regulations*, pp. 341, 344.

15. Ibid., pp. 287, 291.

16. Dyer, p. 65.

17. K. L. Wood-Leigh (ed.), *A Small Household of the 15th Century, Being the Account Book of Munden's Chantry, Bridport* (Manchester, 1956).

18. Ibid., p. xxi.

19. Dyer, p. 212.

20. Ibid., p. 159.

21. D. Gurney, 'Extracts from the Household and Privy Purse Accounts of the Lestranges of Hunstanton, 1519–1578', *Archaeologia* 25 (1834), pp. 422, 445–6.

22. W. Shakespeare, *The Merry Wives of Windsor*, I. iv. 93.

23. *Regulations . . . of Henry Algernon Percy*, pp. 102–3.

24. C. A. Sneyd (ed.), *A Relation, or rather a True Account of the Island of England . . . about the year 1500* (Camden Soc. 37, 1847), p. 25.

25. Heal, p. 159.

26. Ibid., p. 162.

27. H. Best, *Rural Economy in Yorkshire in 1641, being the Farming and Account Books of Henry Best of Elmswell . . .* (Surtees Society pubs 33, 1857), p. 104.

28. G. Scott Thomson, *Life in a Noble Household, 1641–1700* (London, 1937), p. 149.

29. *Collection of Ordinances and Regulations*, pp. 287, 291.

30. T. Webster, *An Encyclopaedia of Domestic Economy* (London, 1844), p. 327.

31. A. L. Cust, *Chronicles of Erthig on the Dyke* (London, 1914), I, pp. 360–1.
32. Mrs W. Parkes, *Domestic Duties*, 2nd edn (London, 1825), p. 117.
33. Webster, p. 327.
34. *Collection of Ordinances and Regulations*, pp. 33, 36, *et passim*.
35. *A Treatise on the Use and Abuse of the Second Table, commonly called the Steward's Table* (London, c.1750), pp. 16–17.
36. M. Waterson, *The Servants' Hall: A Domestic History of Erddig* (London, 1980), p. 82.
37. *A Treatise on the Use and Abuse of the Second Table*, p. 44.
38. J. J. Hecht, *The Domestic Servant in Eighteenth-century England* (London, 1980), p. 113, quoting *The Fortunate Blue-Coat Boy* (1770), I, 97–8.
39. Ibid., p. 112, citing Baker, *James Brydges, First Duke of Chandos*, p. 177. Defoe wrote of Canons, 'No nobleman in England and very few in Europe lives in greater splendour . . . As to house expenses, not less than one hundred and twenty in family (i.e. servants) and yet a face of plenty appears in every part of it . . . every servant in the house is made easy, and his life comfortable. (D. Defoe, *A Tour through the Whole Island of Great Britain, 1725*, new edn (London, 1927), I, p. 388.)
40. *A Treatise on the Use and Abuse of the Second Table*, pp. 29–30.
41. Erddig MS 1542 (62–63) in E. L. Pettitt, *Clwyd Archives Cookbook* (Hawarden, 1980), p. 23.
42. Lady Grisell Baillie, *The Household Book, 1692–1735*, ed. R. Scott-Moncrieff (Edinburgh, 1911), pp. 279–80, 275.
43. *The Housekeeper's Oracle* (London, 1829), p. 143.
44. Parkes, p. 116.
45. T. Jaine, 'Food and the Fortescues', unpublished typescript, p. 7.
46. P. Horn, *The Rise and Fall of the Victorian Servant* (Dublin, 1975), p. 94.
47. A. M. W. Stirling, *Annals of a Yorkshire House* (London, 1911), II, p. 59, note.
48. Baillie, p. 278.
49. Webster, p. 326.
50. Hecht, p. 223, quoting T. Alcock, *Observations on the Defects of the Poor Laws* (London, 1752), p. 48.
51. Horn, p. 8.
52. *A New System of Practical Domestic Economy*, 3rd edn (London, 1823), p. 66; cf. Webster, p. 326.
53. I. Beeton, *The Book of Household Management* (London, 1861), p. 8.
54. Webster, p. 326.
55. *A Treatise on the Use and Abuse of the Second Table*, p. 67; Hecht, pp. 110–11, 130.
56. Stirling, II, pp. 58–9.
57. Cust, II, pp. 84–5.
58. Horn, pp. 101–2; cf. Jaine, p. 7, at a New Year's Day meal laid on in the coach-house for 'our labourers and their wives'.

C. ANNE WILSON

59. Horn, p. 102.
60. Hecht, pp. 128–9; Horn, pp. 102–3.
61. D. Marshall, *The English Domestic Servant in History* (Historical Association, G. 13, 1949), p. 25, quoting J. Woodforde, *Diary of a Country Parson*, 7 May 1792.

4.

Navy Blues:
The Sailor's Diet, 1530–1830

JENNIFER STEAD

While meals in Britain underwent fundamental changes, especially after 1700, meals for the ordinary seaman aboard British navy ships remained virtually unchanged from the Middle Ages to the mid-nineteenth century, depending as they did on three basic items: preserved meat, beer, and ship's biscuit. Difficulties with the preservation of food, and storage on shipboard, were the main reasons for the sailor's limited variety; but his legendary conservative tastes were also to blame, since the British sailor was notorious in resisting attempts to tamper with his customary diet. Until the late fifteenth century this limited diet had nevertheless been adequate, since ships would venture only so far as the beer lasted (usually short voyages of three or four weeks) and they were never too far from land. However, in the Age of Discovery, beginning about 1490, voyages lasting up to eight months or more, for example to America, brought new problems since ships could be at sea for six months without landing. Foods rotted on account of the damp and heat, and became inedible. Biscuit and dried peas were infested with weevils; salt pork or beef, if it had not been carefully prepared, stank and hardened, fats went rancid; beer went sour and water putrified so that hunger, thirst, and deficiency diseases, together with infections, decimated ships' crews by as much as two-thirds.

Nevertheless, the official allowances for each man were generous. In 1545 these were (to be issued at sea as soon as **The Sixteenth Century** the fresh meat and bread were used up): 1 lb biscuit and 1 gallon of beer (eight wine pints) daily, with 1 lb meat four days a week, and on the other three days cheese and dried stock fish. In May 1586 the naval victualler Edward Baeshe had a budget of 4½d per day per man in port, and 5d per day per man at sea. For this he issued the usual items, plus butter, and he doubled the meat allowance. These generous rations attracted many land labourers into the navy: three meals a day, mostly hot, was much better fare than that which most labourers enjoyed on land – 8 lb of salt beef per man per week was almost unimaginable bounty to a poor labourer who rarely ate meat at all. However, these rations were not always issued in full, especially on long voyages and during hostilities, or if the purser suffered losses through storms or rotting supplies; furthermore, corrupt officials cheated the men of both food and pay.[1]

It seems that too often the men, who ate in messes of six, would be given food for only four, called 'six upon four'. The grievances of the Elizabethan sailor were encapsulated by the mutineers on the *Golden Lion* sailing on Drake's Cadiz voyage in 1587, who petitioned their captain

> to weigh us like men, and let us not be spoiled for want of food, for our allowance is so small we are not able to live any longer on it; for whenas three or four men were wont to take a charge in hand, now ten at the least, by reason of our weak victualling and filthy drink, is scarce able to discharge it, and yet groweth weaker and weaker . . . For what is a piece of beef of half a pound among four men to dinner, or half a dried stockfish for four days in the week, and nothing else to help withal, yea, we have help, a little beveridge [diluted wine] worse than pump water. We were pressed by Her Majesty to have her allowance, and not to be thus dealt withal; you make no men of us, but beasts.[2]

For the next 200 years, the major cause of mutinies was to be bad food rather than deficient pay or harsh conditions.

In the summer of 1588 when Queen Elizabeth I's navy was stuck in harbour for many weeks waiting for the Spanish Armada to attack, men on the overcrowded ships suffered great hardships from bad and insufficient supplies. After the battle in July, when the English ships were pursuing the Armada, stocks of food, water, and clothing were exhausted, and the sailors were in appalling condition. Sir Thomas Heneage was told that when the fleet returned from Scotland 'they were driven to such extremity for lack of meat, as it is reported . . . that my Lord Admiral was driven to eat beans, and some to drink their own water'. Throughout the reign, thousands of mariners died 'by the corruption as well of drink as of meat'.[3]

The dreadful hardships on board and extremely hard physical labour made good nourishing food a necessity. Sailors wore their own clothes, if they had any, many were semi-naked and barefoot in all weathers on an unheated ship, most slept on deck, were constantly wet and cold on extremely long watches; often with cold food to eat and no hot drinks. Shivering increases the metabolic rate by 50 per cent; therefore in these conditions they would need the 4,000–4,500 calories their daily allowance (in theory) gave them, and also a high protein intake. (Crews on modern sailing ships, being warmer, need only 3,200 calories a day.[4])

A 'new' disease appeared at this time which was to decimate thousands of seamen until the end of the eighteenth century: scurvy at sea. It had not appeared on short voyages, and it had not affected the long voyages of the Vikings who ventured as far as America because they carried cloudberries and cranberries which keep well and retain vitamin C. It had not been encountered in ships of Mediterranean countries where long journeys were not undertaken. It appeared to be a disease mainly of northern European maritime nations, especially Britain, and so it was thought that fog and cold were implicated. At first it was believed to be infectious. Those ships which set off in spring, after a winter in which no vegetables were eaten, began losing their crews to scurvy in only a few weeks.

By the late sixteenth century the English had learned from the Dutch how to treat land scurvy with scurvy grass, brooklime, cress, and strawberry leaves. However, fresh herbs would not keep at sea; and anyway sea scurvy was thought to be a worse form, caused or exacerbated by salt air and salt food. Sir Richard Hawkins, who had been a prisoner of the Spanish for several years in the Netherlands, had discovered a remedy from his captors: he made it known in 1593 that 'sowre Oranges and Lemons' were an effective antidote to scurvy, though he also gave emphasis to other remedies. In 1601 the English East India Company on its first voyages to the East, put in at Madagascar to pick up 'oranges and lemons of which we made good store of water [juice], which is the best remedy against scurvy'. Efforts were made from the 1590s to preserve the juice by evaporation, but because of the difficulties and expense, and the idea that its curative property was the acid taste, cheaper substitutes such as vinegar and oil of vitriol (sulphuric acid) were used instead.[5]

Serious attempts were made to improve the preservation of food and drink for long voyages. A new method was developed of potting foods, especially meats and fish, under a thick layer of fat. More and more fruits were preserved with sugar, and vegetables were pickled in salt with verjuice, vinegar, or wine. But whereas these all contributed to the varied diet of the officers and gentlemen on board, the ordinary seaman's diet remained basic and monotonous. However, men of enterprise and with a view to profit, such as Sir Hugh Plat, aimed to remedy this. Between 1589 and 1607 Plat promoted a food then unknown in England, pasta, especially macaroni, as an excellent substitute for biscuit and beef on shipboard, as it was light, dry, cheap, and kept well; heat did not rot it 'which is the principal destroyer of sea victuall'. In his puffing broadsheet, Plat also mentioned a method of preserving water, wine, beer, cider, perry, ale, vinegar, or medicine sweet for two to four years by a 'philosophical fire' (possibly alcohol), which also preserved lemon juice, 'because it hath of late been found . . . to be an assured remedy in the scurby'.[6]

In a late sixteenth-century galleon, food was cooked for 400 men in a brick-lined cook-room (later called the galley) situated in the hold, in front of the mainmast. A massive 45-gallon pot was hung over an open fire. By the early seventeenth century the galley was moved to the gun deck near the foremast, and remained in this position even on the first steamships in the early nineteenth century. The term 'mess' appeared at this time to describe the number of men eating from a board which was slung on ropes with a mess stool either side. The men took turns to act as mess-cook, fetching both 'raw' rations and cooked food, and preparing, carving, and serving it.[7]

The Seventeenth Century

In the seventeenth century the British sailor's food was actually worse than that provided a century earlier, partly because the novelty of the new routes and lands was wearing thin, and so there were now no gentlemen adventurers on board to finance extra good victualling; and partly because preservation techniques did not significantly improve. But the main reason was that the navy was neglected. The navy suffered under James I because of corrupt administration and poor leadership, and under Charles I because all attention was centred at home on the fight for civil liberties.

On paper, the diet remained much as it had been before, and though the weekly 8 lb of salt meat was reduced to 6 lb, this was still much more than the Dutch sailor's allowance of only 2¼ lb. But in reality the men were cheated by the corruption and decadence of officers, from Lord Howard of Effingham downwards; for example Sir James Bagg, 'Bottomless Bagg', made a fortune out of the Victualling Office, and there were commissions of inquiry into the running of the Office in 1608, 1618, and 1628. Under the

Commonwealth there was a slight improvement, but at the Restoration Pepys revealed that some of the old corrupt practices had crept back.

In the time of James I, Sir Walter Raleigh said that bad victualling was the main reason why 'they go with great grudging to serve in His Majesty's ships, as it were to be slaves in the galleys'. Captain Sir Ferdinand Gorges, founder of New Plymouth, said of the early Stuart ships 'that some provisions put aboard them is neither fit nor wholesome for man to live on'. Sir Henry Mervyn, commanding in the Downs in 1629, said 'Foul winter weather, naked bodies and empty bellies make the men voice the King's service worse than a galley slavery.'[8] There was serious cheating by government contractors:

> The brewers have gotten the art to sophisticate beer
> with broom instead of hops, and ashes instead of
> malt, and to make it look more lively to pickle it with
> salt water, so that while it is new it shall seem worthy
> of praise, but in one month, wax worse than stinking
> water.

Careless preparation of beef issued to the Ship Money fleet in 1635 caused it to be so tainted that 'the scent all over the ship is enough to breed contagion'. In 1653 complaints were made of the 'unwholesome and stinking victuals, whereby many of them [sailors] are become sick and unserviceable, and many are dead'. John Hollond, in his second discourse on the Navy, 'The Navy Ript and Ransackt' wrote (c.1659):

> For the men will, and do run away rather than eat it,
> and those that do [and] are forced to stay contract
> diseases, sickness, and oft times death by eating it,
> whereby they are either thrown overboard, or turned
> ashore, to the great disservice of the state.

74

In 1695 William Hodges said that for every man who died in action, ten died because of bad or insufficient food.[9] Nathaniel Boteler, writing in 1634, said that navy food was 'a foul cosenage and desperate abuse', and he set out the men's grievances in an imaginary dialogue between a captain and an admiral, in which it becomes clear that there was plenty of bread and meat on the king's ships, but the men were defrauded of it. The captain says:

> I have more than once found sometimes twenty,
> sometimes thirty of the common mariners . . .
> waiting at my cabin door at a dinner time, with their
> beef and pork in their hands, to let me see how small
> the pieces were.[10]

In a publication of 1700 'a sailor' described the victualling as 'the lowest and most corrupt Office of the Navy'.[11] Edward Barlow complained in the 1660s that

> We had but fourteen ounces to the pound, the other
> two being allowed to the purser of the ship for
> scraping of the cheese and butter and dust in the
> bread; yet it was always served out to us without
> scraping, the foul and the clean together, and the
> rotten with the sound, and mouldy and stinking and
> all together.

However, he said that the food was worse on a merchantman and even worse on a Dutch East Indiaman: 'Our English ships commonly make shorter passages and are better provided with provisions not so old.' Merchant ships were sometimes so full of freight that there was no room for water, and the poor sailors were 'whipt at the Geers for drinking the water that is allow'd for the Hogs'.[12]

The unhealthiness of salt meat, which, to make matters worse was boiled in sea water, was a frequent cause of concern. In 1699 'An English Sailor' wrote:

It is of so violent and corroding a Nature, that the
Honble *Robert Boyle* Esq; has so prepar'd it, as to
make it dissolve Iron Bars: but perhaps the victualler
thinks the Sailors Bodies more durable than Iron.[13]

Salt beef for shipboard was not hung and dried, as on land,
but left in salt, in barrels, sometimes for five or six years, so
that it became inedible. Many ideas were put forward from
the sixteenth century onwards for preserving meat unsalted.[14]
In 1709 'Barnaby Slush', a 'sea-cook', in a publication setting
out the sailors' grievances, suggested that because of its
intolerable saltiness the beef should be steamed, as practised
by some British and Dutch merchantmen, to draw the brine
out. He also mentioned queues of twenty or thirty men
waiting at the captain's cabin door to show him their tiny
pieces of meat, and urged that the men be given 3 lb of their
supposed 4 lb of meat on fleshdays, and that they be given
their full ration of peas, instead of the half ration which the
purser often gave, 'for Peas is a Noble Food'.

Oatmeal, which on land at this time had begun to be
despised, except in the north and Wales, was thoroughly
disliked by all but northern and Welsh sailors. Slush wrote
'this *North Britain* Diet . . . Burgoo . . . they fairly toss it
over Board, at the Gun-ports, as fit only for hogs'.[15]
However, it had once been well liked. Gervase Markham
wrote in 1631:

if a man be at Sea in any long Travel, he cannot eat a
more wholesome and pleasant meat than these whole
Greets boyled in water till they burst: and then mixt
with Butter, and so eaten with Spoons, which
although Seamen call it simply by the name Loblolly,
yet there is not any meat, how magnificent soever the
name be, that is more toothsome or wholesome . . .[16]

Barnaby Slush stressed the importance of alcohol to the sailor: wine, rum, beer 'is their all in all; the very Cement that keeps a *Mariners* Body and Soul together; insomuch that a Tar sets as high a Regard on a single Quart of Ship Beer, as his whole Days Allowance in Provisions'.[17]

The British seaman's entrenched conservatism in food habits, especially his love of meat, prevented the introduction of a more healthy variety. Boteler's captain thought the British should eat like the Spanish and Italians who both on land and at sea 'live most upon rice, oatmeal, biscake, figs, olives, oil and the like; or at least like the French and Dutch, who content themselves with far less portion of flesh and fish than we do, and instead thereof do make up their meals with peas, beans, wheat [flour], butter, cheese, and those white meats as they are called'. He advocated the use, when abroad, of potatoes, plantains, oranges, lemons, and limes 'which are excellent against the Scorbute'. But the admiral replied 'Our seamen are so besotted in their beef and pork that they had rather adventure on all the calentures [fevers] and scarbots [scurvies] in the world than be weaned from their customary diet, or the least bit of it.' The captain deplored the fact that, when on foreign shores, the English sailor rejected healthy but strange fruits and vegetables, and instead hunted for animals to turn into salt meat, such as turtles and wild 'beeves'.[18] Pepys also condemned the conservatism of the sailor: 'Seamen love their bellies above anything else', and to provide inadequate or disagreeable food 'will render them disgusted with the King's service sooner than any other hardship'.[19]

The men's hunger was made worse by the sight of the officers' well-fed livestock on board: hogs, sheep, goats, geese, turkeys, ducks, hens.[20] Officers' fare was described by Henry Teonge, who made two voyages in the Mediterranean as ship's chaplain. The first was an expedition in 1675 against the Barbary States. Teonge loved the good cheer and life at sea; the slightest pretext caused the punch bowl, wine, and spirits to be brought out, and every Saturday night was spent in drinking bumpers to wives, sweethearts, and absent friends. The officers' ordinary fare was very good. On 13 November 1678, on the way to Almeria:

> We had an aitchbone of good beef and cabbage; a
> hind-quarter of mutton and turnips; a hog's head and
> haslett roasted; three tarts, three plates of apples, two
> sorts of excellent cheese: this is our short-commons
> at sea.

However, the officers' fare when visiting foreign ports or when entertaining foreign visitors on board was lavish, and Teonge describes several gargantuan feasts. This was in great contrast to the men's diet; their beef bought in Cyprus by the niggardly purser was bad and was flung overboard, and they had to eat dry bread instead. Two seamen who had stolen a piece or two of beef were ordered to be tied to the mainmast with the raw beef round their necks, their mouths rubbed with it for two hours by the other seamen.[21]

Scurvy was still decimating the navy, for the advice on citrus juice was officially disregarded. In their ignorance of the real nature of scurvy, the Admiralty and most merchant companies still chose to provide their surgeons' cupboards with the cheaper alternative of oil of vitriol. Citrus juice was carried only by a few individual captains who were convinced of its usefulness, such as Captain James Lancaster, who as a consequence lost none of his men to scurvy on the *Dragon*, on one of the first voyages to the East by the newly formed East India Company in 1605.[22] Beer was thought to be anti-scorbutic since it was noted that scurvy started only when the beer was used up; but another drink, cider, actually was slightly anti-scorbutic. Cider had been known as an excellent shipboard drink from the sixteenth century, even though it was then often of poor quality. In the seventeenth century, production methods in England were improved, and juice pressed from sound apples was fermented into a

78

fine wine. Cider kept as well as wine, and much better than beer or ale. The sailors drank it diluted with ship's water, whereupon it was called 'beveridge' which just means 'weak drink', and could be made from either wine or cider. William Clowes, the Elizabethan surgeon, said beveridge was the sailor's best drink against scurvy. However, the Admiralty did not make official issue of cider, even though its medicinal value seems to have been well known.[23]

Attempts were made to find ways of preserving drinking water. From about 1635 Samuel Hartlib was at the centre of a circle of *cognoscenti* (later to form the Royal Society). He collected many ideas from correspondents on every aspect of knowledge, including some on how to make stinking waters sweet for shipboard; but none of these remedies was effective. Hartlib noted that the answer seemed to be not to drink water at all – for on Dutch East India ships Dutch sailors drank wine rather than water and did not die so soon as the British sailors.[24]

In 1667 the amount of meat in the sailors' rations was restored to 8 lb per week; on voyages south of latitude 39°N, instead of beer, they were to have a quart of wine or a pint of brandy; instead of meat, they were to have flour, suet, and raisins (for pudding); and instead of fish and butter, rice and oil.[25] Pepys attempted to improve the quality of supplies. In the victualling contract drawn up by him on 31 December 1677 each man was to have daily 1 lb of 'good, sweet, sound, well-baked, and well-conditioned wheaten biscuit', 1 gallon, wine measure, of beer, 'brewed with good malt, and very good hops, and of sufficient strength', 2 lb of beef 'killed and made up with salt in England' (there was a prejudice against Irish beef) for Sundays, Mondays, Tuesdays, and Thursdays; 'or, instead of beef, for two of those days, 1 lb of bacon or salted English pork and a pint of pease'. On Wednesdays, Fridays, and Saturdays, besides bread and beer, each man was to have either:

⅛ part of a full-sized North Sea cod of 24 in. long; or
⅙ part of a haberdine [salt, or wind-dried cod], 22 in.
long; or ¼ part of a haberdine, 16 in. long; or 1 lb
avoirdupois of well-savoured Poor John [salted or
dried hake]; 2 ounces of butter; 4 ounces of Suffolk
cheese or ⅔ of that weight of Cheddar.

However, in the absence of an efficient system of inspection
and control, the quality of shipboard rations did not
improve.[26]

**The Eighteenth
Century**

In the eighteenth century, navy rations remained largely the
same as before. For example, in 1745 the allowances were
(besides the daily gallon of beer and 1 lb of biscuit): Sunday
and Thursday, 1 lb salt pork and ½ lb peas; Tuesday and
Saturday 2 lb salt beef; Monday, Wednesday, and Friday, 1
pint oats, 2 oz. butter, and 4 oz. cheese, with ½ lb peas
extra on Friday. So on three meatless days (called Banyan
days, after an Indian vegetarian sect), the men got nothing
but biscuit, beer, buttered groats, and cheese, unless they
managed to save meat from the day before.[27]

Biscuit, called pilot bread, hard tack, or pusser's nuts, was
made from stoneground wholewheat flour and so was a
good source of fibre and calories; each man got four 4 oz.
biscuits per day. These were round, with a depression in the
middle, and of an adamantine hardness. Corrupt victuallers
sometimes adulterated them with peaflour and bone dust.
They were packed in bags and soon became damp and
musty, and were attacked by maggots and weevils, which
softened them.[28] Tobias Smollett in *Roderick Random* wrote
that 'every biscuit . . . like a piece of clock-work, moved by
its own internal impulse, occasioned by the myriads of
insects that dwelt within it'. The sailors nicknamed the
Deptford yard where biscuit, peas, and flour were put up,
'Old Weevil'.[29]

Biscuit was usually so hard that it had to be soaked in
water before use, and then it could be fried with salt pork

fat, or mixed with salt pork and vinegar, in a dish called skillygolee or lobscouse. Any scraps of chance fresh meat, fish, or vegetables were added, onions being a favourite, and after 1750, potatoes; it was eaten with a spoon. If made without meat it was breadscouse or blindscouse.[30] Lobscouse and figgy dowdy were promised to lads as an inducement to volunteer (1807). Biscuit could also be bashed to crumbs in a bag with a marlin spike, and either baked with chopped meat or made into a cake with pork fat and sugar. For breakfast 'Scotch coffee' could be made with burned biscuit boiled to a thick paste, then sweetened with sugar; this seems to have been a crude version of 'toast and water'.[31]

Salt meat preservation was still unreliable.[32] The meat could be as hard and dark as old mahogany, and was sometimes carved by the seamen into ornamental boxes. At sea it was still impossible to soak the salt out properly before use, and often it raised blisters on the tongue; the meat also lost half its weight on boiling.[33] In Smollett's *Roderick Random* (1748) the boy Roderick, who had just been pressganged, watches Thomson, who has befriended him, make a dish of salmagundy, it seems with raw salt beef:

> Ordering the boy to bring a piece of salt beef from
> the brine [he] cut off a slice and mixed it with an
> equal quantity of onions, which seasoning with a
> moderate proportion of pepper and salt, he brought it
> into a consistence of oil and vinegar. Then tasting
> the dish, assured us it was the best salmagundy that
> he had ever made.

Roderick tastes it: 'No sooner had I swallowed a mouthful than I thought my entrails were scorched.'[34]

Salt pork with dried peas was called dogsbody. Peas were liked, though Roderick Random is shocked to find that on meatless days peas constitute the entire dinner:

We heard the boatswain pipe to dinner, and immediately the boy belonging to our mess ran to the locker, from whence he carried off a large wooden platter, and in a few minutes returned with it full of boiled peas, crying, 'Scaldings,' all the way as he came. The [table] cloth, consisting of a piece of old sail, was instantly laid, covered with three plates, which, by the colour, I could with difficulty discern to be metal, and as many spoons of the same composition, two of which were curtailed in the handles, and the other abridged in the lip. Mr Morgan himself enriched this mess with a lump of salt butter, scooped from an old gallipot, and a handful of onions shorn, with some pounded pepper. I was not very much tempted with the appearance of this dish.[35]

No pots, pans, or cutlery were supplied for ordinary seamen until the 1890s. In the eighteenth century the ordinary seaman's mess was supplied only with a wooden bread-barge (in shape a truncated cone), a vinegar barrico (small cask), and an oval tub for fetching and carrying food.[36]

Cheese for shipboard was traditionally tough Suffolk skim-milk cheese, which was pressed hard to make it keep better, and nicknamed Suffolk bang or Suffolk thump.[37] If it was cured incorrectly it could become either so hard that it was impossible to eat, or too soft and corruptible. During the Seven Years' War the Suffolk suppliers, on account of the urgent and greater demand, cut the curing time, and the cheese rotted and stank. Hailes wrote to Rodney in 1758 that the cheese might 'by its nauseous smell, be liable to cause an infection', and Anson complained that most of the cheese on board his squadron was inedible. As a result of the serious and universal complaint, the long-standing Suffolk monopoly was ended in 1758. Cheshire, Gloucester and Warwickshire cheeses were provided instead, which were more expensive and more subject to decay; however,

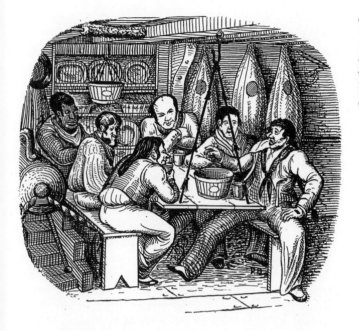

6.
Sailors' mess table
slung between two
guns on the
gundeck, 1815.
Drawing by
P. Brears after
George Cruikshank.

complaints noticeably decreased.[38] Butter was just as
difficult to preserve; olive oil would have been a much
better alternative. Butter, salted in casks, went rancid, and,
in a hot ship, ran to oil and was used for greasing the ship's
rigging blocks.[39]

Oatmeal or whole oats, groats, made into loblolly were
generally unpopular; they were apt to be full of weevils, and
badly cooked, so that one surgeon said: 'it was cruel to
expect the men to eat [them]'. However, they were obviously
liked by one sailor in the 1770s, who, being a good singer
and therefore popular, visited every mess 'where a
pandoodle, a bowl of burgo, or a dish of scratch-platter was
to be given'. (The name burgoo took precedence over the
name loblolly sometime before 1750.[40]) Sometimes, saved
gobbets of salt meat were put into this dish, and after 1805
molasses was served with it.[41]

Vinegar was an important condiment, and was desperately needed to make dull, often cold, food interesting. It was used as a disinfectant, and was also thought to be anti-scorbutic because of its sharp taste. However, pickled fruit and vegetables were actually anti-scorbutic because small amounts of vitamin C were preserved in the acid. In 1758 Henry Jackson mentioned 'the prodigious Consumption of Pickles in the Navy'.[42]

As in previous centuries, water on ships was unfit to drink; it was used mainly as permanent ballast in the bottom tier of casks in the hold, and was used as a drink only in emergencies. Various methods of preserving fresh water were tried, notably by Stephen Hales. Some of these were: the addition of slaked lime and sulphur; distillation; filtration through charcoal; and 'ventilation', the blowing of air through water with bellows. However, none of these was practicable or successful.[43] In 1733 Captain Cook supplied fresh water by melting sea-ice (when sea water freezes, it distills). In 1762 James Lind advocated distilling sea water by fitting still heads or musket barrels to boiling coppers to draw off and evaporate the steam, but this did not produce large amounts. Bad water was a continuing difficulty. In 1812 the water aboard one ship was described as 'like the extract of ditches around Sheerness'[44] – until the problem was solved by the advent of steamships, for their iron storage tanks were hygienic and capacious, and periods at sea now lasted no longer than two or three weeks. An efficient method of distilling sea water was introduced about 1850.

The importance of alcohol nutritionally cannot be over-emphasised, since the sailor obtained by far the most of his daily calories from it. His daily 8 wine pints of beer supplied almost half as many calories again as his 1 lb biscuit, and far more than his meat, butter, cheese, peas, or oatmeal; and so the quality was very important. Properly made strong beer would last for a year, but the navy's beer put aboard a hot ship in summer went sour or 'sweated' very quickly, and the pitching and tossing made it deteriorate even more quickly. It was no wonder that the men made the most of being in home port, where they were allowed to drink more than their usual allowance once visitors were on board, and great drunkenness ensued.[45] In long voyages and in foreign places the men drank watered wine in the proportion of 1 measure of wine to 8 of water, or watered spirits – 1 measure of spirits to 16 of water.[46] This did not disguise the taste of putrid water but the slight anti-bacterial property of wine would have lessened any harmful effects if the mixture were allowed to stand. The sailor's favourite drink in the seventeenth and eighteenth centuries was flip – a mix of beer and spirit, often brandy, sweetened with sugar and heated with a hot iron – also called Sir Cloudsley, in memory of Sir Cloudsley Shovel (1650–1707), who was very fond of it. Ned Ward wrote of the 'honest tar': 'his darling liquor is Flip, which makes him as fat as a porpoise and as valiant as Scanderburg'. There was nothing so comforting as a 'small chirping Can of Flip'. Flip seems to have been the sailor's only warm drink until the introduction of cocoa about 1800. Bumbo was a mixture of rum, water, sugar, and nutmeg.[47]

Rum, a by-product of British West Indian sugar production, had been introduced in the mid-seventeenth century, and was issued neat to the crew; it was general issue by 1721. A state of almost perpetual inebriation helped them tolerate the hardships on board. However, this became a problem, and in 1740, in order to drive 'that Dragon Drunkenness out of the Fleet' Admiral Vernon, commanding the fleet in the West Indies, inaugurated the diluting of the rum ration. His nickname was 'Old Grog' because of the grosgrain cloak he always wore, and the drink became known as grog. The daily half pint (8 oz.) which is a large mugful, was to be diluted with two pints of water, and issued, not all at once, but twice a day. This was done to the order 'Up spirits', and the drink was served out while a fiddler played a lively tune. Occasionally, however, too many sailors were still groggy during afternoon watch, so weaker 'six-water' or 'seven-water' grog was issued by subsequent officers. However, drunkenness still occurred because the men could save up their grog, or sell it to others. Under Nelson the daily grog, issued once a day at noon, was 1 gill rum in 3 gills water with lemon juice and sugar. Drunkenness continued, so in 1804 grog was replaced by tea, but Bonaparte was threatening invasion, and the switch to tea caused 'murmuring in the fleet which was frightful at such a moment'; so grog was restored. In 1825 grog was reduced yet again to ¼ pint twice a day 'without disturbance or complaint'.[48]

In 1793 tea for convalescents was introduced by the surgeon of HMS *Pandora*. Cocoa became the first official hot drink issued to all sailors, and not just convalescent ones. Dr Trotter welcomed it:

> In a cold country it could be singularly beneficial;
> what a comfortable meal would a cup of warm cocoa
> be to a sailor in a winter cruise on the North Sea or
> the Channel, on coming from a wet deck on a rainy
> morning watch.

In 1824 the allowances included 1 oz. cocoa, ¼ oz. tea, 1½ oz. sugar daily, while oatmeal was reduced to ½ pint per week.[49]

Victualling began to be urgently reviewed during the wars of the mid-eighteenth century, when the fighting force of the navy was continually and seriously weakened by illness and death. As a result of serious complaints by Boscawen, Hawke, and Anson, the Victualling Board started to dismiss private contractors and cheating officials in order to process more and more foods in the navy's own yards, and to control standards.[50] However, complaints from the men continued. In 1761 William Thompson said that mariners had frequently put their day's ration of salt meat into their tobacco boxes (they frequently got only 10 oz. to the lb), that they had 'made *buttons* for their *Jackets* and

Trowses, with the *Cheese*', and that 'Carpenters . . . have
made *Trucks* to their Ships flagstaffs with *whole Cheeses*,
which have *stood* the *Weather equally with any timber*'.
The flour was weevilly, musty, and rock solid; the biscuit
was contaminated with other substances and full of maggots;
the beer 'stunk as abominably as the foul stagnant water
which is pumped out of many cellars in London at midnight'
– the men had to hold their noses to drink it, and they threw
the pork and burgoo out of the portholes, even though they
were cruelly punished if discovered.[51] Some spoilage was
inevitable in damp warm storage conditions, where mites,
insects, and rats were ineradicable, and when barrels crashed
and split. Most stores were deep in the airless and
unventilated hold, and kept directly above the insanitary
ballast of wet sand and shingle. However, spoiled food was
often served out to the men so that the purser would not
make a loss.

The purser joined the navy for a profitable career; he was
in charge of the massive provisioning of the food, drink,
and clothes which he had to guarantee with his personal
finances. He was responsible for every pennyworth consumed, and where there were losses and wastage, he had to
claw back what he could by reducing the men's rations. He
was allowed to take one-eighth of every man's allowance.
Consequently, a purser's pint was only 14 oz., and beer was
served by the 'purser's quart'; if the entire ship was rationed
by two-thirds, called 'six upon four', that is food for four had
to stretch to feed six, he was supposed to pay the men
compensating 'pinch-gut money'. Albatrosses following
ships were said by the sailors to be pursers' ghosts searching
for their old ships to make up their losses. These losses
could be heavy through bad weather, shipwreck, or looting
by pirates or the enemy. The purser had to keep very
complicated accounts, to log every man's food consumption
for every single day. This was further complicated because
the men need not fetch their ration, which meant they were
owed it, or need only fetch part, they could take unused

provisions back, they could exchange items for some other one, or could sell their allowance for grog, and each month they could change their messes.[52] One of the main causes of the 1797 mutiny was that sailors felt cheated of their food. They petitioned that 'our provisions be raised to the weight of sixteen ounces to the pound, and of better quality'. They also requested not to be served flour in British held ports, and asked that 'there might be granted a sufficient quantity of vegetables . . . which we grievously complain and lay under want of'.[53]

The navy supplied live cattle to furnish fresh meat for as long as possible, but animals often died in storms, and fodder and dung were problems. Anyone who could afford it could bring livestock (with the first lieutenant's permission) such as pigs, sheep and poultry.[54] Goats were kept for milk (usually only for officers) and were allowed to roam and scavenge, but were unpopular when they ate the sailors' bread which hung in bags in each mess. The officers appointed one of their number to be 'mess caterer' for that voyage, to whom they all paid a contribution, and who was responsible for buying in the extras. The captain lived in his own quarters with his own servants, his own cook, livestock and supplies.

In the early eighteenth-century ship's galley, food was cooked in a huge 'copper' let into a brick hearth, but from the 1750s cooking was done in an enclosed iron stove.[55] Most food was boiled, but baking and roasting could be done on a small scale for officers, or for the sick. Occasionally the ship's fires had to be put out, for example, during stormy weather, when the enemy was sighted, or when a hot climate dried all the ship above water; and then the meals were dreadful indeed – raw salt pork or beef, cheese, and biscuit. In the 1790s the men, many of whom had been on watch since 4.00 a.m., had breakfast at 8.00 a.m., grog and dinner at noon, and at 4.00 p.m. supper: usually biscuit and butter or whatever food they had saved, plus grog or wine. Officers had breakfast at 8.00 a.m., dinner at 2.00 p.m., supper at 6.00 p.m., and punch at 9.00 p.m.[56]

Private provisions brought from home or shore did not last very long. Four weeks after setting sail from Lymington in 1798, Lady Hunter, sailing to Gibraltar on a ship with 1,000 men on board wrote: 'the mess stock is all finished, all very sorry for themselves, nothing to eat but their rashers of salt meat and ships biscuits'.[57] When ships were moored some distance from the shore, extra food could be bought from the bumboats which carried the filth from ship to shore, and returned with fresh fruit, vegetables, bread, liquor, and other supplies. In foreign ports, where sailors disliked substitutes (for example, oil instead of butter, and yams, flour, chick peas, maize, or rice instead of bread), they might buy more pleasing alternatives. At sea the men caught fish or seabirds. Other supplements such as rodents were not so appealing, for, even when starving, many English sailors baulked at eating rats (whereas the French ate rats happily). W. Richardson, writing in 1792 about his time in the brig *Active* at Calcutta, said the ship was alive with rats:

> One of our people used to skin, grill and eat them and they tasted as well as a rabbit. Had I known as much then as since I would have had many a good meal of them, for our diet on board here was nothing but rice, dhal, ghee and water.[58]

In the eighteenth century, scurvy and epidemics continued to affect seriously the manning of the navy, especially during the War of Jenkins' Ear, the War of Austrian Succession, and the Seven Years' War. Lind's famous *Treatise of the Scurvy* appeared in 1752, in which he proved that citrus juice, fresh vegetables, and fruit were incontrovertibly curative; and yet the Admiralty chose to ignore this most vital advice. However, from 1756, frightened by the losses of manpower through disease and death, they did begin to issue fresh meat and vegetables, which made possible the lengthy blockades in the Mediterranean and in Canadian waters which ultimately won the Seven Years' War. Novelties such as malt, sauerkraut, and portable soup were issued for medical comforts.[59] During the American War of Independence the supply of vegetables lapsed, and scurvy may have cost Britain the American colonies. Dr Thomas Trotter urged the renewed supply of vegetables and in 1796 50 lb of greens for every 100 men was issued, with the consequence that Nelson's navy was healthier than any that had gone before it.[60] Lemon juice, preserved by Lind's method of gentle evaporation, was not made official issue for all until 1795, a whole forty-two years after Lind's important treatise, during which thousands of seamen needlessly died of scurvy. This date marked a turning-point in naval history. The juice was issued after six weeks at sea at the rate of 1 oz. per day, and was usually mixed with the noon grog. 'Of all the means which defeated Napoleon, lemon juice and the carronade gun were the most important.' The merchant navy did not officially issue it until this was enforced in 1844. About 1850 the navy was persuaded to substitute West Indian limes, which were cheaper than the Mediterranean variety, but with deleterious results, as these only had half the vitamin C content.[61] From this practice came the American term for British sailors – 'limeys'.

An important innovation in the sailor's diet was the introduction of tinned meat.[62] In 1817, Donkin, Hall and Gamble supplied the British navy with tinned meats in place of portable soup as a medical comfort. They proved especially useful in voyages of exploration and surveying, and in 1847 tinned meat was made general issue.[63] Biscuit remained a staple until the First World War, when it was made in dog biscuit factories.

It is interesting to consider that, because of the nature of the victualling, the British navy was dogged by deficiency diseases until the end of the eighteenth century; but degenerative diseases did not figure then, partly because the sailor's diet was rich in fibre. However, the modern navy, in spite of its unprecedented choice of foods, is also plagued by nutritional deficiencies, which lead to degenerative diseases, because personnel choose to eat foods which are low in fibre, high in fat and sugar, and lacking vitamins B and C. In the 1970s the number of deaths from these diseases in the armed forces was among the highest of any group in Britain.[64]

Notes and References

1. Navy pay was lower than it had been in the Middle Ages. In 1546 sailors earned 6*s* 8*d* a month; in 1585 this was raised to 10*s* a month. It was not usually the amount of pay, but the delay in payment which caused dissatisfaction. Christopher C. Lloyd, *The British Seaman* (London, 1968), pp. 42, 43, 48; Robert W. Kenny, *Elizabeth's Admiral* (Maryland, 1970), p. 40; C. Ernest Fayle, *A Short History of the World's Shipping Industry* (London, 1933), pp. 163, 180.
2. Charles N. Robinson, *The British Tar in Fact and Fiction*, 2nd edn (London and New York, 1911), p. 54; Lloyd (1968), pp. 49, 50.
3. For grievances of the Elizabethan mariner, see *The Naval Tracts of Sir W. Monson*, ed. with a commentary by M. Oppenheim, 5 vols, (London, Navy Records Society, 1902-14); Lloyd (1968), p. 42; H. W. Hodges and E. A. Hughes (eds), *Select Naval Documents* (London, 1936), p. 17; Kenny, p. 154; Malcolm Thick, 'Sir Hugh Plat's Promotion of Pasta as a Victual for Seamen', *Petits Propos Culinaires* 40 (1992), p. 46.
4. J. Watt, E. J. Freeman, and W. F. Bynum (eds), *Starving Sailors: The Influence of Nutrition upon Naval and Maritime History* (Greenwich, National Maritime Museum, 1981), p. 199.
5. John Woodall, surgeon to the East India Company, wrote about scurvy in *The Surgeon's Mate* (1617): 'The vse of iuyce of Lemons is a precious medicine, and wel tried [or] vse oyle of Vitrioll . . . an especiall good medicine in the cure of scuruy.' Sir John C. Drummond and A. Wilbraham, *The Englishman's Food* (London, 1939), pp. 162, 166, 168-9, 172; Lloyd (1968), p. 68; Thomas McLachlan, 'History of Food Processing', *Progress in Food and Nutrition Science* 1 (1975), p. 464; Sir Hugh Plat, *The Jewel House of Art and Nature* (London, 1653), p. 180.
6. Plat claimed he introduced pasta to the navy, and that in 1596 Sir Francis Drake took it on his voyage. In 1595 Hawkins wrote that he had taken a new 'kind of victuells for sea service devised by Mr. Hughe Platte': Thick, pp. 43, 47. Sir Hugh Plat, *Certaine Philosophical Preparations of Foode and Beverage for Sea-men, in their long voyages* (1607). I am grateful to C. Anne Wilson for suggesting the philosophical fire could have been alcohol.
7. Una A. Robertson, *Mariners' Mealtimes and Other Daily Details of*

Life on Board a Sailing Warship (The Unicorn Preservation Society, Edinburgh 1979), p. 12.

8. Fayle, p. 166; Lloyd (1968), pp. 50, 52, 58, 59, 71.

9. Lloyd (1968), p. 62. *Complaints of Seamen*: Kendall to Admiralty Commissioners, 13 July 1653 (Navy Records Society, 41, p. 275, quoted in Hodges and Hughes, p. 68; J. Hollond, *Two Discourses of the Navy, 1638 and 1652*, ed. J. R. Tanner (Navy Records Society, 7, 1894), Second Discourse chapter iii, quoted in Robinson, p. 69.

10. *Boteler's Dialogues*, ed. W. G. Perrin (Navy Records Society, 65, 1929), p. 56.

11. *Remarks on the Present Condition of the Navy, and particularly of the Victualling . . . in a Letter from a Sailor* (London, 1700), p. 14.

12. Lloyd (1968), p. 108; William Hodges, *Humble Proposals for the Relief, Encouragement, Security and Happiness of the Loyal, Courageous Seamen of England* (London, 1695), p. 45.

13. *Boteler's Dialogues*, p. 65; *The State of the Navy consider'd in relation to the Victualling by an English Sailor*, 2nd edn (London, 1699), p. 11.

14. Sir Cheney Culpeper wrote to Samuel Hartlib about 'A special matter to powder bief for ships in the Spring February et March especially for at other months it will take no salt'. Also Wheeler wrote to Hartlib: 'I doe promise to shew a way how to cause beef to keep above a year that when they do come to make use of it they will have beef not onely good to eate boyled but will be as fresh that they can make good broth for the officers and soldiers aboard.' Hartlib Ephemerides 54/33/1A, 2A, Sheffield University.

15. Barnaby Slush (pseud.), *The Navy Royal; or a Sea Cook turn'd projector* (London, 1709), pp. 34, 66, 67, 68.

16. Gervase Markham, *The English House-wife*, 4th edn (London, 1631), p. 242. This opinion of buttered oats was repeated by Richard Bradley in his edition of Noel Chomel's *Dictionnaire Oeconomique* (London, 1725), 2 vols, under the entry 'Oatmeal'.

17. Slush, p. 71. French sailors also would rather go without food than wine, see Watt, Freeman, and Bynum, p. 73.

18. *Boteler's Dialogues*, pp. 65, 67; Fayle, p. 178; Lloyd (1968), p. 57. Robinson, pp. 94–5.

19. N. A. M. Rodger, *The Wooden World: An Anatomy of the Georgian Navy* (London, 1986), p. 82; Lloyd (1968), p. 94.

20. Slush, p. 71.

21. *The Diary of Henry Teonge 1675–1679*, ed. with an introduction by G. E. Manwaring (London, 1927), pp. 39, 138, 206, 228.

22. Lloyd (1968), p. 68; R. K. French, *The History and Virtues of Cyder* (New York and London, 1982), p. 58.

23. Francis Bacon, who in 1618 became Lord Chancellor to James I, wrote: 'Cider and Perry are notable beverages in Sea voyages' and in *New Atlantis* he wrote that cider and oranges were 'an assured remedy for the sickness taken at sea'. In John Evelyn's *Pomona* (p. 28) there is a letter which says cider is 'specifically sovereign

against the scorbut' and in 1676 John Worlidge said the same. French, pp. 14, 28, 52, 59, 60, 61. John Parkinson, in *Paradisi in Sole Paradisus Terrestris* (1629) wrote: 'Yea, many Hogsheads and Tunnes [of cider] are made especially to be carried to the Sea in long voyages, and is found by experience to be of excellent use, to mix with water for beverage' (p. 589).

24. A note to Hartlib dated 10 November 1635 mentions a new oven invented by Dr Kufler, which, besides cooking, has 'an art of turning salt water into fresh which with the other is wondrous profitable in ships'. Boiling the water was believed to kill its vital spirit and make it putrefy sooner; also, fuel was limited. The Spaniards were probably the first Western Europeans to distil water at sea, as can be seen in the records of Dr Andrés de Lagunn in 1566. Other suggestions for purifying water were to sink an empty wax-sealed cask in the sea (Aristotle (*Meteorologia* 2, 3) had said that water would filter through the wax which would prove to be drinkable); to filter sea water through charcoal or sand (Boteler, p. 59); to add 1 lb powdered brimstone (sulphur) to each hogshead (Platt, *Jewel-house*, p. 8).

25. Lloyd (1968), p. 95.

26. The term 'poor John' is an indication that, on land, dried fish had already become despised. At sea, dried fish was kept in a special dry room. Teonge, p. 22.

27. Rodger, p. 83; Drummond and Wilbraham p. 302.

28. Watt, Freeman, and Bynum, p. 30; *Remarks on the Present Condition of the Navy . . . from a Sailor* (1700), p. 14; Robertson (1979), p. 23, 26. In the seventeenth century the Dutch discovered that if packed in airtight boxes and kept dry, biscuit would keep perfectly well. See Robert Boyle, *Some Considerations touching the Usefulness of Experimental Naturall Philosophy* (London, 1663), part II, p. 107. By 1800 biscuit was kept on British ships in special bread rooms, lined with tin, the air kept dry with pendant stoves.

29. T. Smollett, *Roderick Random* (London, 1748), ch. 33. Weevils consumed the wheat germ; weevils tasted bitter and made the throat feel dry. Maggots with black heads, 'bargemen', felt cold as one swallowed them. Robertson (1979), p. 28; Watt, Freeman, and Bynum, pp. 11, 30.

30. Robertson (1979), p. 24; Lloyd (1968), p. 208. Made by many north European sailors, lobscouse was a shipboard dish of some antiquity. It was probably originally lapscouse – lapskuis in Lapland included walrus; Swedish Lapskojs is still made with salted meat; German labskaus often includes meat and herrings together. Returning sailors brought the dish home, and it was widely known in England until the nineteenth century, surviving later only in the stew-loving north. A dweller in Liverpool is still called 'scouse' after the widespread eating of lobscouse by the sailors and dock workers.

31. Robertson (1979), p. 23. For toast and water, see Helen M. Pollard, 'A Liquid Diet', in *Liquid Nourishment*, ed. C. Anne

Wilson (Edinburgh, 1993), pp. 52–4.

32. It was difficult to salt meat in hot weather, and in cold weather blood stayed in the carcasses and spoiled the pickle. A sloppy method of pickling pork for the navy was simply to throw freshly killed pork into barrels of heavily salted water, and since the blood and lymph stayed in the brine, it created off-flavours. This was called 'barrel-pork' or 'sea-junk' (junk was the term for old rotted rope). Stephen F. Gradish, *The Manning of the British Navy during the Seven Years' War*, Royal Historical Society (London, 1980), pp. 152–3; Dorothy Hartley, *Food in England* (London, 1954), p. 327.

33. Fayle, p. 180; Una A. Robertson, '"Mariners' Mealtimes": The Introduction of Tinned Food into the Diet of the Royal Navy', *Food Conservation* (London, 1988), p. 149; Gradish, p. 143.

34. *Roderick Random*, ch. 26. Tobias Smollett was a surgeon's mate in 1741 on the Carthagena expedition, which is described in the novel.

35. Smollett, ch. 25.

36. Robertson (1979), p. 10.

37. Richard Bradley wrote that these Suffolk cheeses 'will bear transporting through the hottest Climates, which the more tender-made cheeses will not without corrupting, unless they are put into Oil'. *The Country House-wife and Lady's Director* (1736), I, p. 75.

38. Gradish, pp. 147–8; Rodger, p. 85.

39. Watt, Freeman, and Bynum, p. 10.

40. William Ellis, *The Country Housewife's Family Companion* (London, 1750), p. 206. The nickname 'loblolly boy' remained for the surgeon's mate, who was derided as knowing very little about the business of a seaman. Robinson, p. 298; C. Lloyd, J. Keevil, and J. L. S. Coulter, *Medicine and the Navy, 1200–1900*, III (London, 1961), p. 85; Robertson (1979), p. 149.

41. Robinson, p. 282; Lloyd and Coulter, pp. 83, 85; Robertson, p. 24.

42. Henry Jackson, *An Essay on Bread* (London, 1758), quoted in Drummond and Wilbraham, p. 234. Pickled walnuts especially were a good source of vitamin C, but onions also, containing 10 mg of vitamin C per 100 g, would supply minute but valuable amounts: only 10 mg per day are needed to stave off the worst effects of scurvy.

43. Royal Society of London, *Philosophical Transactions from 1665–1800*, vols 1–90 abridged with notes by Charles Hutton, George Shaw, Richard Pearson (London, 1809), vol. 48, 1753, p. 551, vol. 49, 1744, pp. 635–43, vol. 50, 1758, pp. 243–5.

44. *Five Naval Journals, 1789–1817* (London, Navy Records Society, 1951); see under the Rev. Edward Mangin, 1812, p. 13.

45. Watt, Freeman, and Bynum, p. 31; Gradish, pp. 154–6; W. H. Long, *Naval Yarns 1616–1831* (London, 1899), p. 120; Rodger, p. 92.

46. Rodger, p. 92, n. 17.

47. Edward Ward, *The Wooden World Dissected* (London, 1707),

p. 92; Slush, p. 28; Smollett, ch. 34.

48. Watt, Freeman, and Bynum, pp. 10, 14, 31. Grog could be made with any spirit, for example, arrack, a spirit made from practically anything, such as dates or rice.

49. Watt, Freeman, and Bynum, pp. 9, 13; Robertson (1979), p. 19.

50. Gradish, pp. 144–9.

51. William Thompson, *An Appeal to the Public to prevent the Navy of England being supplied with pernicious Provisions* (London, 1761), pp. 17–21. There was even more wastage in the French navy because of the dishonesty of supply officers. The French navy had massive stores in the 1760s and 1780s, but these went bad, causing illness, death, and reduced manoeuvres. Their salt beef was especially poor. If they captured a British man-of-war, they would eat British salt beef in preference to their own. Watt, Freeman, and Bynum, pp. 74, 75, 83.

52. Rodger, pp. 89–94.

53. Ibid., p. 314.

54. Not many officers or petty officers now took their own livestock, 'and seldom carry any other thing to sea, on a cruise, than a few pieces of corned beef, a bag or two of potatoes and some onions'. The Hon. John Cochrane, *The Seaman's Guide: Showing how to Live Comfortably at Sea* (London, 1797), quoted in Robertson (1979), p. 43; Rodger, pp. 70–1.

55. The Brodie cast-iron fire-hearth was introduced in 1781 with an oven that could bake bread in 80 lb batches, plus a condenser to provide a little distilled water. Robertson (1979), p. 12.

56. Robertson (1979), pp. 4, 5, 53.

57. *The Journal of General Sir Martin Hunter* (Edinburgh, 1894), p. 117.

58. Rats taste 'something between a frog and a rabbit', wrote Henry Labouchère, quoted in Julian Street, *Table Topics* (London, 1961), p. 136. About the same time as Richardson, Baron Jeffrey Raigersfeld wrote that during the night, the captain of the hold would 'fish' in the hold with bait and catch four or five rats and have them skinned and cleaned and ready for sale next morning. As they had fed on cheese and biscuits, their flavour when grilled and peppered was good. Eating fresh rats regularly would stave off advanced scurvy since rats can synthesise vitamin C. In actuality, rats were probably eaten more frequently than has been thought, since the ordinary sailor's subculture was largely unknown to the writers of records, who were usually officers. (Watt, Freeman, and Bynum, pp. 29, 30.)

59. Portable soup – squares of condensed gelatine and stock – were issued generally from 1757 to supplement peas and oatmeal. Sauerkraut, an idea taken from the Dutch, was thought by Dr Thomas Trotter 'very trifling' as an anti-scorbutic; even so in 1782 2 lb per week was issued to all seamen, who characteristically resisted it at first. Watt, Freeman, and Bynum, pp. 12, 13, 29; Drummond and Wilbraham, p. 318; Gradish, p. 159.

60. Watt, Freeman, and Bynum, p. 12.
61. Drummond and Wilbraham, p. 320; Watt, Freeman, and Bynum, pp. 13, 24.
62. Bottled and tinned foods, being neither dried nor salted, were regarded as fresh, and therefore good for the scurvy. A novel method of preserving roast beef, in tin canisters, invented by the Dutch for use on shipboard, was described by Captain Stedman in the 1770s. In 1795 the Frenchman Nicolas Appert experimented with bottling foods; in 1810 he published his methods, and within ten years factories were set up in Europe and America. *Naval Review*, 27 (1939), p. 103; McLachlan, p. 468.
63. Donkin and Hall of Dartford copied onto their tins from Appert the words *'boeuf bouilli'*, which became 'bully beef'. Stuart Thorne, *The History of Food Preservation* (Kirkby Lonsdale, 1986), pp. 25–7.
64. Watt, Freeman, and Bynum, p. 45.

5.

School Dinners – Style Louis XIV

LYNETTE MUIR

Mme de Maintenon, morganatic wife of King Louis XIV of France, was always interested in education. Even before her rise to favour in the 1680s, when she was still Widow Scarron, she had been helping a small school at Rueil for girls of all classes, run by an Ursuline nun called Mme de Brinon.

Sometime after the Queen's death in 1684 Mme de Maintenon (as she had become) was married to Louis in a secret ceremony. The school was moved to larger premises at Neuilly; then, in 1686, Madame persuaded the king to found a school specifically for the daughters of the impoverished nobility who had suffered badly in the wars. There was already a number of schools for their sons. The king agreed and in 1686 the Royal Foundation of Our Lady and St Louis was built on the edge of the village of St Cyr, about 2 km from the Palace at Versailles. It is probably the oldest purpose-built girls' school in Europe.

The building, which is still in use as a cadet school for the French army, was designed by Jules Hardouin Mansart, the royal architect, and was completed in a very few months because the king was eager to get the project going. The layout of the interior was planned by Mme de Maintenon herself with the help of Manseau, her steward, and Nanon Balbien, her *femme de chambre*.

Most of our information about the *temporel*, or practical side, of St Cyr comes from Manseau's *Mémoires*, which he began to write in 1689 for a 'Lady' who had asked for them.

After her death he continued them for his own children. The memoirs cover the period from the founding of the school in 1686 to the end of 1692, and give many details of the building and equipping of the school. They are our main source of information for the provision, serving, and cost of the meals for the community.[1]

Other details are taken from the memoirs of the school compiled over the whole century of its existence by the Dames de St Cyr.[2] A separate document drawn up in 1750 gives a detailed account of the daily routine that can be compared to that given by Manseau seventy years before.[3]

There are also the hundreds of letters and *discours* written by Mme de Maintenon herself.[4] Particularly useful for the cost of living is a letter written by Madame (as she was always, if improperly, called at St Cyr) to her brother in 1678, when he married (against her advice) and settled in Paris. His wife was young and foolish, so Madame sets out a detailed list of the food needed for each day with its costs and quantities, and works out for him a monthly and annual expenditure for all his household needs (including the carriages and the opera!) that will give him a comfortable life within his income. It is worth remembering that Madame herself had been very poor most of her life and knew the value of economy and good management.

The community at St Cyr consisted of 250 *demoiselles* divided into four classes indicated by their coloured ribbons: red for ages 7–10; green for 11–13; yellow for 14–16; and blue for 17–20. The criteria for admission were poverty, four degrees of nobility, and a certificate of good health. When they reached 20 years the girls had to leave, and, if they had not opted for the religious life or had a marriage arranged for them, they went home to their parents. It was Madame's hope that the girls so trained would improve the quality of family life of the French nobility, and especially the upbringing and education of their children.

The Dames de Saint Louis, who were the teaching and administrative staff, numbered thirty-six when they were at

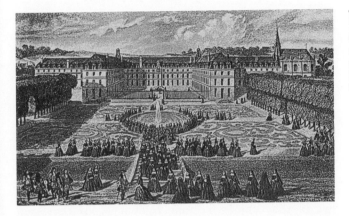

7.
The School for
Girls at St Cyr,
near Versailles,
probably the oldest
purpose-built girls'
school in Europe.

full strength. The community was completed by forty lay sisters, who looked after most of the household work with the help of the girls themselves and a number of paid servants. Although the king was very insistent that St Cyr was not a Convent, the Dames and the lay-sisters were professed religious and never left the Enclosure, the main residential area of the Foundation.

In the outer court lived the priests and the male members of the community; other men on the payroll (but probably not resident) included a doctor, a surgeon, a cobbler, and a man to look after the school clock. (Since the day was organised on a strict time basis his job was important.)

Daily Routine and Meals at St Cyr

The *demoiselles* rose at 6 a.m. and, after dressing, went down to the *demoiselles'* refectory, outside which were copper basins and faucets, where they washed their hands and rinsed their mouths. This was the only fresh direct water supply in the school apart from the kitchen quarters. The original site was chosen partly for its very good springs, which should have supplied St Cyr but which were contaminated because of the damage done to the site during the building of the school. Mansart sited the building too low on the slope of the ground, and they always had problems

99

with flooded cellars. Madame never forgave Mansart and blamed him for the fevers and epidemics which caused the death of 300 girls during the century of its existence. 'He may have fooled the King'; she remarked once, 'he has never fooled me.' Drinking water therefore had to be brought from the aqueduct originally constructed to carry water to the royal menagerie situated in the park halfway between St Cyr and the Palace of Versailles. The school water was pumped in by horse-driven pump. (The provision of water cost £500 a year according to the accounts. It is not clear whether the water for the sluices to the privies or for washing the kitchen court whose runnels were cleaned out twice a week came by the pump from the aqueduct or from the springs.)

Having completed their limited toilet, the girls then had breakfast – a piece of good bread. It was always white. Madame said the Dames might eat brown if need arose, but the girls must always have white if possible. This rule was broken only in the serious famine years of the early 1700s. The 1750 memoir adds that in winter the girls had *pain au lait*, which might be a type of bread or of bread and milk, or *des croutes au pot* (sops in broth). These were probably not part of the original menu. Breakfast was followed by Mass and the morning lessons.

At 11.00 a.m. the girls went to the *demoiselles'* refectory for dinner. The Dames and lay-sisters ate separately, except for those supervising or serving. From the beginning the dinner consisted of *un potage, un bouilli, une entrée et des fruits. Potage* at that date was a very thick mixture of vegetables cooked with meat – something like a stew except that the meat or fowl was whole, not cut up. Madame's letter to her brother refers to *une volaille bouillie sur le potage*, a fowl boiled on the *potage*. *Bouilli* was the meat broth made by simmering meat for a very long time. Except in Lent (see below) the *entrée* was roast meat, usually beef or mutton. Madame insisted that the girls should have plenty of meat. The day's ration was ¾ lb for the junior classes, reds and greens, and 1 lb for the seniors. The meal was completed by milk in summer, and by salad and fruit, depending on the season.

In her letter to her brother Mme de Maintenon allows 15 lb of meat and two pieces of roast for twelve people per day. (His household included several menservants.) Two kinds of meat are mentioned both in the memoirs and the letter: *viande* and *rosti*. The former appears to be a general term and probably means the meat used to make *potage* and *bouilli* etc., while the *rosti* (or *rostisserie* – Manseau uses both terms) was bought by the piece, ready cooked. The same practice is found in households in Paris and Versailles generally. Apparently only the royal kitchen at Versailles, the Grand Commun, which fed thousands of people every day, was big enough to have its own roasting spits and ovens. There is no reference to them at St Cyr (see below).

The afternoon brought recreation and more lessons. Then at 3.00 p.m. the girls had collation, which again was white bread served in the classrooms. Any girl who wanted a drink was taken down to the refectory. The girls never drank anything but water.

Supper at 6.00 p.m. was similar to dinner, but the meat was mainly poultry or game birds and there was only one bowl of soup with it.

The girls went to bed at 9.00 p.m.

The Building and Food Service

In order to make clear Manseau's description of the preparation and serving of the meals, I should explain that the school building was in the form of a huge 'H' shape with a cross piece about 650 ft wide running west to east, divided into equal thirds by two uprights about 360 ft long running north to south. The building was of a uniform width of 30 ft inside.

The *cour des cuisines*, with the blue classroom and dormitory over the main kitchen, was in the south-east corner of the cross formed by the main residential area of the Enclosure: the Dames were members of a religious

8.

Plan of the school
at St Cyr, based
upon a drawing by
Le Sieur Delorme
of 1688.

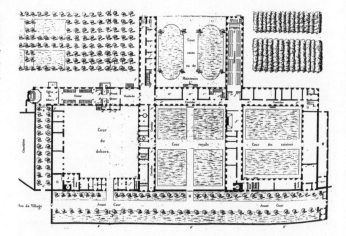

8.

Plan of the school
at St Cyr, based
upon a drawing by
Le Sieur Delorme
of 1688.

order and could not go outside this Enclosure, even to the
outer courtyard. The dining room was the north arm with
the yellow class above; the reds were on the east and the
greens on the west.

Manseau drew scale plans of the different floors of the
buildings with coloured-in beds etc. to show which room
was which. The water supply by the refectory and in the
kitchens are also coloured in a light blue. The plans have
numbers for the rooms and items in them and an
accompanying commentary. Unfortunately, the original
plans are A1 size and the reproduction in the only printed
edition of Manseau is octavo, so it is virtually impossible to
read the numbers. However, it is clear that the *cour des
cuisines* included the following rooms: the kitchen and
storerooms for the infirmaries were on the south side of the
court; on the east were two large wood stores, one for
faggots and one for corded wood. The apothecary's rooms,
including a laboratory with apparatus for distilling, a special
water supply with portable conduit, and a room with stone
sinks for washing herbs, are on the north.

The main kitchen was on the west side, with the
storerooms. These included one for oil and other things of

102

this kind. There was also a *fruiterie*, fitted with sloping shelves with a rim, on which the fruit was stored; a bread store, near the refectory; a *garde-manger*, or general larder, with cupboards and hooks. A room with a bread-oven included for emergencies was used meanwhile as a storeroom (the members of the community could not have baked in the *boulangerie* in the outer court, as it was outside the Enclosure).

One location I cannot explain is the *potagers en retour*, which is on Manseau's plan. *Potagers* can be pot-herbs so that is no problem; but *en retour* usually means in exchange. However, *des retours* is used for goods brought back on a ship's return voyage, so it might have been some kind of reciprocal arrangement with the local farmers, a bit like a tithe or similar obligation given in return for land – hence, a storeroom for such supplies.

The room with stone sinks was dedicated to washing '*herbes*' – vegetables and salads – and a scullery which contained a wooden, lead-trimmed cistern with taps which discharged water into stone sinks was used for washing the pots and pans. In the dispensary they kept spare kitchen equipment and the candle chest.

The *grande cuisine* was situated at the north end of the wing nearest to the refectory. Since the school was purpose-built and the type of food to be served was known from the beginning, Manseau planned and equipped the kitchens to deal with it. There were five *fourneaux* (stoves for boiling or stewing), one for the *marmite* of each class and one for the Dames, and one *four* or bake-oven. Food for the staff and priests attached to the community who lived in the outer courtyard beyond the enclosure was also provided from the main kitchens (except for a short period in 1688), but Manseau never explains where the cooking was done for them. The lay-sisters probably ate the *restes* (leftovers) from the Dames or the *demoiselles*.

Each of the five *fourneaux* had its own pans, cauldrons, and equipment of all kinds marked with the name or colour of the group for whom it was intended. Particularly in the early days Madame kept a strict eye on this, and on all aspects of the arrangements as Manseau explains: 'There was not a meal served when she was at St Cyr that she did not visit the kitchens and the refectory, tasting everything to make sure it was good. . . . sometimes I have seen her remain in the kitchen for several hours to get the cooks in the habit of working properly.'

Mme de Maintenon was most insistent that the food should be not merely adequate and properly served, but hot – no mean task when serving 250 girls at a sitting. The refectory was a long room (30 ft wide by about 150 ft long) with rows of fixed tables and benches down each side on raised wooden steps. There are four pairs of tables marked on each side in the plan. The floor of the room was tiled. The girls sat in class order, younger in front and older behind 'as they sat in church', says Manseau. The memoir of 1750 tells us that the greens sat in front of the yellows and the reds in front of the blues, nearest the Dame presiding who sat on a small dais at the far end. A picture of the Crucifixion hung on the wall opposite a lectern for the reader, who was usually one of the elite group of senior girls who wore black ribbons. In 1750, but not on Manseau's plan, there is a special table at one end of the refectory for the blacks.

Pottery bowls and plates were set in front of each girl (all marked with the school crest and class colours when they were made), and the cold food, milk or salad and fruit, was set out beforehand. Then the lay-sisters carried in the *barques* – long stretchers with short legs and covered with white linen cloths – on which were two dishes of meat or soup for each class (all marked). The cooked meat was arranged in portions on dishes which were kept warmly covered on the *fourneaux* in the kitchen.

The girls whose turn it was then helped to serve. The pewter dishes were specially made to Manseau's own design, round, with handles at each end, and shaped on one side like a barber's basin so the girls could hold them against the white aprons which covered their brown woollen dresses. One girl held the dish while another, armed with a silver spoon and fork as long as the ones used in the kitchen, served out the portions. Thus, Manseau claims, they could distribute the food quickly and so quietly that not a word of the reading was lost. In the 1750 memoir, however, we are told that the Dame presiding over the meal had a bell which she rang to stop the reader while the next course was being served. It was also her responsibility to look out for those girls who were hearty eaters and make sure they got large portions.

There is a location marked on Manseau's plan called the *passage des portions* near the north end of the kitchen wing. It seems likely that this was a way through under the so-called *demoiselles'* staircase (which led to the classrooms above) by which the portions of meat, etc. were carried through from the kitchens as quickly as possible.

At first the girls did not have forks, only spoons and knives because Mme de Maintenon did not want to put the king to the extra expense. (As it was, the table silver, including dishes, goblets, spoons, and forks for the Dames and goblets and spoons for the girls, came to more than £5000.) The girls' dishes were pewter, but silver forks at more than £8 a piece were provided for them by Madame at her own cost in April 1688. The girls also had napkins, which were kept in the 250 drawers in the tables.

In Lent, when, of course, no meat could be eaten at all, great pains were taken to prevent the food seeming dull. At Mme de Maintenon's request, Manseau prepared lists of provisions needed for each day for the *dépensier* (manciple): 'In them I put the quality and quantity of everything they would serve at each table both for dinner and collation beginning on Ash Wednesday. Noting that the same dish should never be served two days running and that the classes should have different food so that by changing round in this way they might the more easily put up with

Lenten fare (*viandes maigres*).' Unfortunately, this Book of Instructions, which was bound and kept in the *dépensier's* office for use in future years, has not survived.

The Food Supply The supply of food for this large community was carefully organised by the ubiquitous Manseau. As soon as the school was founded, tenders were invited from the purveyors, and the cheapest were given the orders. However, a strict eye was kept on the quality of the basic foodstuffs provided, and poor quality goods were rejected.

When Manseau eventually gave up the job of running the *temporel* in 1688 and a full-time steward was appointed, Manseau drew up one of his usual detailed memoranda: *Instructions pour le sieur de la Ferté* . . . etc. Among La Ferté's duties, Manseau included checking the quality and quantity of the supplies provided in wine, corn, and meat, as well as smaller items. The wine was presumably for the outside members of the household, including the priests (and possibly the Mass wine), as neither the girls nor the Dames drank it.

At first, bread was supplied by the Minister of War, Louvois, who had it baked by the bakers of the *Invalides* (the French equivalent of the Royal Hospital at Chelsea), recently founded by the king. The school provided the ovens and other necessary equipment (the *boulangerie* was sited in the outer courtyard), and the best wheat in France; from this he provided bread at the rate of 180 lb of good white bread for each *sétier* (approximately 4.2 bushels) of wheat. All the leftovers from the milling, etc. belonged to him.

At the end of the first year it was recognised that he was making a huge profit on the contract, and it was decided to have the bread baked in-house. The community bought the wheat, and had it ground and supplied daily to the baker. Since we do not have a wages list after the first year we do not know how much he was paid. The bran flour left over after the fine sifting of the white flour was given to the local poor. (They also received the other leftover food, except the best portions which went to the infirmary, presumably because the numbers there were small and they could use up a modest amount of food.)

The steward's instructions give us a clear picture of the running of the bakery:

> You will choose the grain of prescribed quality, have it stirred up in the *greniers* [granaries] and measured at the same time and will deliver it to the baker. You will keep the keys of the *greniers* and will take care that the bran and the groats are not left in the flour and that the aforementioned grain is not changed at the mill. You will have the bread weighed in the morning and carried to the tower [the entrance to the Enclosure] at the prescribed time. You will keep a list of the amount delivered which can be compared with that kept by the Dames to ensure perfect order. [p. 95]

At first eggs and butter were provided by a friend of the Superior, Mme de Brinon. This *'demoiselle'*, who had four sisters in the house, had her home in the Vexin region, and was commissioned to send dairy produce each week from her region. For this she received a pension of £200 a year, since Mme de Brinon claimed that the butter and eggs supplied thus would be better and at a more proper price. Manseau makes it quite clear that he disapproves of this arrangement, and indeed his general dislike of Mme de Brinon comes over throughout the book in little remarks. For example, he tells us that in addition to her own daily portions (which she ate in her apartment and not in the Dames' refectory) she received also two pieces of *rosti*, so she could either send it to those she thought needed extra, or feed the many guests she had. (Mme de Maintenon, who to begin with had complete faith in this Superior, wanted her to be able to do everything she liked, and had obtained a special dispensation for her to receive people in the Enclosure.) Manseau also particularly disliked her habit of having food cooked in her anteroom on a charcoal stove which he claimed (but strictly only in his private memoirs) was ruinous to the fine parquet floor!

However, one of her ideas that Mme de Maintenon had always resisted was that the school should keep its own poultry or its own farm animals of any kind, since she said it was not economic and they had neither the space nor the time to make such a project viable. The farms belonging to the community, from which they drew part of their income, presumably supplied them with milk.

Although Manseau and Nanon Balbien had a difficult time for eighteen months between the demands of Mme de Brinon and their own duties to their adored Mme de Maintenon, it was Manseau who had the last laugh. Mme de Brinon, whose promotion to the post of Superior of St Cyr seems to have gone to her head, finally wore out Madame's patience and was dismissed by a *lettre de cachet* in December 1688.

After her departure the dairy produce was bought from a merchant in Maintenon (the village where Madame had her estate, about 10 miles from Versailles). Eggs and butter were supplied at a fixed price all the year round, and the Dames had the freedom to return any of the weekly delivery that 'was found to be bad'. The butter was used in cooking and the eggs especially for making a liaison to thicken the *potages* and *ragouts*. There is no evidence to suggest that the girls ate eggs hard-boiled, though they may have done so. It is well known that they were a favourite delicacy of the king.

As steward, La Ferté also had to check the deliveries made by the butcher, the *rostisseur*, and the *patissier*, and presumably also the fruit, vegetables, and spices which were all bought at the prices that had been agreed with the suppliers. Judging by Mme de Maintenon's letter to her brother, the fruit most likely to be eaten were apples (either raw or in a compote with sugar), and pears. Vegetables commonly eaten in Paris at this date include cabbage, beans, dried peas, asparagus, and leeks. Potatoes were rare, but other roots were available. Green peas were a delicacy which would certainly not have been found at St Cyr. There is no clue in the memoirs to the exact vegetables consumed as 'salad'.

There were orchards at St Cyr which probably provided some of their supplies, and there is some indication that part of the 25 *arpens* of garden (about 1½ acres) were given over to the growth of vegetables. When a determined attempt to drain the site was made in 1691, *potagers* (which are kitchen gardens as well as what grows there) were created in the south-east corner between the *cour des cuisines* and the isolation infirmary. The gardener, who was responsible for the upkeep of the gardens, including the quincunx and the flower beds, and for the supply of manure etc., was paid £1,800 a year.

Festivals

The routine of the school food was sometimes varied by special treats, especially for major feast days of the church such as the Assumption or the school's patronal festival of St Louis. This was also the king's name-day and it was the custom, apparently, for the local garden-owners to send him baskets of fruit (of which he was very fond). In a letter written to the Superior, Madame half-jokingly says that the courtiers complain they got no fruit at all for the feast of St Louis last year, as the king sent it all to St Cyr! Holidays were also given for Madame's name-day of St Francis (4 October), and for major French victories or other celebrations.

Sometimes the extras were provided by Mme de Maintenon herself. We have, over the years, references to her presenting baskets of cherries and peaches, boxes of sugared almonds, butter for the afternoon bread, pastries for the girls, and preserves for the Dames. The peaches were apparently eaten out of doors, which seems a prudent move, and suggests that other festive collations might also be taken as a *fête champêtre*. In the hot weather the girls certainly spent a lot of time outside, under the trees at the far end of the gardens.

If the extra was being provided by the school, as on the occasion, for example, of the Superior's installation (she was elected every three years after Mme de Brinon's departure), it seems to have been usually pastries. Mme de Maintenon was insistent that they should be bought and not made at home: 'spending your time with your hands in the dough making flamiches like farmers' wives is not what you have been appointed to do', she told the Dames. On at least one occasion hippocras was served, but it seems to have been only for the Dames and would certainly have gone against the idea that the girls should drink only water. (That they drank wine at home is clear from several comments.)

Manseau's *Rule*, drawn up in 1687 to give the Dames guidance on how to work out their budget, includes an item for *menus extraordinaires*. This would probably include the celebratory food as well as the extra for Mme de Brinon and any visitors who came.

In 1692 the new bishop of Chartres, the St Cyr diocesan, was consecrated in the school church with great celebrations including dinner for a large number of visiting prelates. Four VIP tables were set up, three outside and one (at which Madame presided) inside the Enclosure. There were also ten tables served for the other guests. However, the expense for this was met by Madame personally. (The king, incidentally, though he frequently visited the school never ate there or indeed anywhere but in his own palace.)

La Ferté's job description includes: 'When there are *repas extraordinaires*, you yourself will fetch the provisions, on other days you will send the purveyor off in good time in the morning so that he will be back at the time fixed by the Superior.'

Food for the Sick The infirmaries had their own kitchens and pans and dishes, as well as their own bedding and clothing. There was a dining-room on the ground floor below the *demoiselles'* infirmary where the convalescents ate. The isolation infirmary in a corner of the grounds quite separate from the rest of the buildings presumably had all its own kitchen arrangements, too. We know that much of its furnishing came from the original school at Neuilly.

There is little information to be gleaned on the subject of the food in the infirmary. The patients were given sops dipped in broth for breakfast if they could not eat bread. Manseau mentions *bouilli* for the infirmary, and Madame on one occasion criticises the Infirmarian saying firmly that 'reheated vegetables especially if they have been cooked in butter are not suitable food for invalids'. Another time Madame tells the Infirmarian that she has obtained for her the oranges she wanted for her patients, but reminds her that though oranges taste refreshing 'they have never cured anyone of anything yet'. 'Keep to the quinine' is her constant cry, and she adds that when she was governess to the royal children she told them it was good for them and they drank it down like water without protest.

In a letter she says that she has learned from the Ursuline sisters who came and helped to nurse the girls during an epidemic (mainly caused by the bad water supply and drainage) that salads were bad for invalids. When her brother suffered from haemorrhoids she advised him to eat plenty since it is better to have indigestion than constipation, but to avoid food that is salty, peppery, or sharp (vinegary?). In the course of her life Madame had had a wide experience of illness, and seems to have been a competent and caring nurse who inspired the same feelings in her Dames.

Income and Expenditure

Finally, let us consider what this all cost – and here again some interesting comparisons can be drawn with the letter to Madame's brother. Fortunately, part of Manseau's innumerable duties in the early days was not only keeping the school accounts but teaching the Dames how to do them, and he includes details of them in his memoirs. By

111

piecing things together from a number of years we get quite a full picture.

As is usual in France in the centuries before the Revolution, the money of account is £sd (livres, sous, and deniers), based on the pound *parisis*, which was worth considerably less than the pound sterling. The Foundation's total annual income was £150,000, out of which they were expected to save enough for repairs to buildings as well as giving a dowry of £3,000 to each girl when she left. We learn from one of Madame's talks to the 'blues' that such a sum invested brought in 50 écus a year, which was enough to keep one person in decent if modest comfort. It is important to remember that all the girls came from very poor families, who would not be able to provide dowries for their marriage or for them to enter religious orders, and might not even have enough to live on. The school was completely free; and no kind of presents to the community or school were accepted, except from the king or Madame herself.

During the first part-year of the school, from July to December 1686, the food (*provisions de bouche*) cost only £13,481, which Manseau notes was low because the price of grain and wine was low. At the end of the full year 1687, they found they had fed 332 people at a cost of £40,819, which is worked out by the month and day also, giving 6s 8d per day. In 1689 the daily figure is 6s 6d, and in the accounts of 1692 it was 8s ½d. (Manseau is, of course, a professional accountant, giving his sums to the minutest fractions.) As the Dames had worked out with Manseau's help that they should keep their expenditure on food to £48,000 a year (not including the *menus extraordinaires*) if they were to live within their income, they had done well.

Some detailed prices are available. In 1687 meat was 4 sous per lb, and 23 sous for a piece of roast. (This was good value if we compare it with Mme de Maintenon's list for her brother in which the meat was respectively 5 sous per lb and 25 sous per lb for a piece of roast.) Bacon was 6 sous per pound. Eggs, when bought from the merchant in Maintenon, were £18 per thousand, and butter 8s per lb.

Manseau gives no costs for fruits, etc., but some information can be gathered from the letter in which Madame allocates £1 10s per day for fruit, and suggests that this will supply a pyramid of apples and pears which can be used up gradually and will retain its appearance if fresh leaves are put under it as needed. To make a compote only ¼ lb of sugar is needed, and sugar was 11s per lb. The other spices seem to have been fairly cheap, since they are included among the little extras for which she allows in rounding up her daily figures.

Madame's menu with costs for a day for twelve people is as follows:

15 lb meat at 5s	£3	15s
2 pieces of *rôti*	£2	10s
bread	£1	10s
wine	£2	10s
fruit	£1	10s
wood, candles, and tapers	£2	18s
	£14	13s

This, says Madame, means you can manage on £15 per day, or £500 per month, which includes an allowance for laundry, torches, salt, vinegar, verjuice, spices, and trifles.

I have quoted this daily menu in detail because it reveals how interested Madame was in accounts, and how good a manager she was. It also indicates that the major details of the menus for the girls are those of her own brother's household, i.e. suitable to their rank and financial situation. However, she tells her brother that this allowance of £15 per day should also cover an entrée of sausages on one day or neck of veal or sheep's tongues; also a *potage* with a fowl boiled in it in the morning, and two roast capons with the *rosti* in the evening.

Her brother had ten servants, seven of them men, which

accounts for the large wine bill. She says she has allowed 4*s* worth of wine for each of the four lackeys and two coachmen, because that is what Mme de Montespan gives to hers. When the letter was written, Mme de Maintenon was governess to the king's children by this lady, so she was in a good position to know what she paid. She herself always liked to know how her accounts stood, and took pains to have the Dames taught book-keeping as well as the girls. Jetons or counters were used in all the offices and in the classrooms.

In one of her talks to the 'reds', the youngest girls, Madame drew for them a portrait of the reasonable girl, for reason was Madame's constant guide. To be *raisonnable* was to be good and to be happy. Among the qualities of the reasonable red she lists 'gaiety' and describes her as always doing everything heartily and joyfully:

> Now our reasonable person is in the refectory. What does she do? She eats with a good appetite; not greedily with her head in the plate but elegantly and decently. And since it is God's will that we should find pleasure in eating she does so, simply and without scruple.

From what we know of the school-dinners at St Cyr, that seems to me a very reasonable thing to do.

Notes and References

The only English study of the school at St Cyr is H. C. Barnard, *Madame de Maintenon and Saint-Cyr* (London, 1934, republished 1971).

1. The MS of Manseau's *Mémoires*, with the large coloured plans which he drew up, is preserved at the Bibliothèque Municipale at Versailles. It has been edited only once (with minor omissions) by Achille Taphanel in 1902. The edition was limited to fifty copies. There is no copy available on inter-library loan in England.
2. The MS of the *Mémoires de ce qui s'est passé de plus remarquable depuis l'établissement de la Maison de Saint-Cyr, des commencements jusqu'à l'année 1740*, is also in the library at Versailles. Parts of it

114

were published in 1848 by Théophile Lavallée. (There is a copy in Cambridge University Library but no inter-library loan copy available in England.) Lavallée also wrote the principal study of the school: *Histoire de la maison royale de Saint-Cyr* (Paris, 1853), which includes a later set of plans than those of Manseau, drawn up when the school was being made into a full religious community in 1694–6.

3. The 1750 memoir is preserved in MS in the Bibliothèque nationale and was published for the first time in J. Prévot, *La première institutrice de France: Madame de Maintenon* (Paris, 1981). This is mainly a selection of letters and documents dealing with the teaching and organisation of St Cyr. It does not quote Manseau's memoirs.

4. There have been numerous partial editions of Madame de Maintenon's letters but no definitive one. I have used the *Correspondance générale de Madame de Maintenon*, edited by Lavallée (Paris, 1865–6) and the *Lettres de Madame de Maintenon (1655–1701)*, edited by Marcel Langlois (Paris, 1935–9), vols 2, 3, 4, and 5 (vol 1 was never published). A full list of the editions is given in the bibliography of J. Prévot (see note 3, above).

6.

Bastille Soup and Skilly: Workhouse Food in Yorkshire

PETER BREARS

The cloth was laid in the Workhouse Hall,
The great-coats hung on the white-wash'd wall:
The paupers all were blithe and gay,
Keeping their Christmas holiday,
When the Master he cried with a roguish leer,
'You'll all get fat on your Christmas cheer!'
When one by his looks did seem to say,
'I'll have some more soup on this Christmas-day'
        Oh the Poor Workhouse Boy,

At length, all on us to bed wos sent,
The boy wos missing– in search we went:
We sought him above, we sought him below,
We sought him with faces of grief and woe;
We sought him that hour, we sought him that night;
We sought him in fear, and we sought him in fright,
When a young pauper cried: 'I know we shall
Get jolly well wopt for losing our pal.'
        Oh the Poor Workhouse Boy,

At length the soup copper repairs did need,
The Coppersmith came, and there he seed,
A dollop of bones lay a grizzling there,
In the leg of the breeches the poor boy did wear!
To gain his fill the boy did stoop,
And, dreadful to tell, he was boil'd in the soup!
And we all of us say, and we say it sincere,
That he was push'd in there by an overseer.
        Oh the Poor Workhouse Boy.[1]

Bastille Soup and Skilly

The lines of this Victorian street ballad, together with the potent image of the harsh, depressed life of the workhouse boy presented in Charles Dickens's *Oliver Twist*, now form part of our popular historical culture. However, even today there are many for whom these fictional representations are quite superfluous, for they can remember when the great red-brick union workhouses were seen as the final home for many of their friends and relatives, and potentially for themselves, too. The purpose of this chapter is to examine the food provided in the workhouses of Yorkshire up to the end of the nineteenth century; but first it will be necessary to trace the development of poor relief in general within the county.

The Middle Ages to the End of the Seventeenth Century

During the medieval period, the church (with its numerous monasteries and hospitals), the guilds in the major towns, and all the major householders made substantial provision for the poor. The hospitals might provide long-term residential care for those who were unable to support themselves due to old age or illness, while the wealthier institutions and individuals might employ an almoner to distribute aid to the poor, including the broken food left over from their tables. These works formed an essential part of the Christian's duty, as expressed in the Acts of Corporal Mercy, which are illustrated in the early fifteenth-century windows in York's parish church of All Saints, North Street. Here the good man is seen:

1. Feeding the Hungry;
2. Giving drink to the Thirsty;
3. Entertaining the Stranger;
4. Clothing the Naked;
5. Visiting the Sick; and
6. Relieving those in Prison.

After the Dissolution of the Monasteries, hospitals, and religious gilds in the 1530s provision for the poor continued

117

9.
Oliver Twist asks
for more. This
classic image of
life in the
workhouse was
created by George
Cruikshank to
illustrate Charles
Dickens's great novel
of 1838.

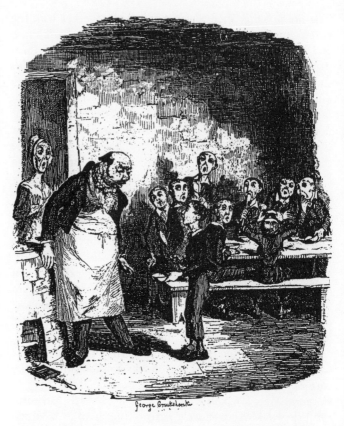

to attract private charity. Over the next 300 years numerous individuals helped the poor by bequeathing land, stocks, and money for their maintenance, as the long, painted benefactors' boards record in many of our parish churches. Others continued to give food to the poor; thus Sir Hugh Cholmley of Whitby recalled how 'Twice a week, a certain number of old people, widows and indigent persons, were served at my gates with bread, and good pottage made of beef, which I mention that those which succeed may follow the example.'[2] Regrettably few of the gentry took his generous approach,

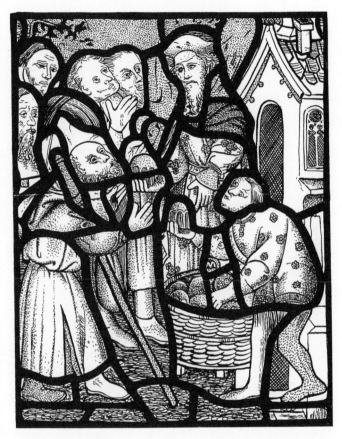

10.
Feeding the poor, one of the six Acts of Corporal Mercy illustrated in the fifteenth-century windows of All Saints Church, North Street, in York. Drawing by P. Brears.

and this traditional form of hospitality gradually passed out of general use.

The social and economic changes brought about by the Dissolution caused a great increase in the number of vagrants, whom the state began at once to control. Earlier legislation had been designed to prevent the poor from moving out of their own locality, but an Act of 1536 provided the first compulsory payments for the relief of the poor.[3] Those who refused to work were successively whipped, had their right ear cropped, were gaoled, and were finally executed as felons and enemies of the commonwealth. An Act of 1547 further permitted such 'sturdy beggars' to be enslaved by anyone who would take them, feed them on bread and water and refuse meat, and force them to work by beating, chaining, or any other means, with execution still remaining as the final solution.[4] These and later sixteenth-century Acts largely failed to stem the increasing numbers of paupers, although they did provide a working framework within which local government could begin to tackle the problem. They required, for example, that every city, corporate town, and parish should keep a book recording the names of all householders and the impotent poor, and also appoint two collectors of alms for the poor every Whitsuntide.[5]

In the city of York, this legislation was quickly implemented and measures were taken to make it as effective as possible. On 9 February 1588, the corporation decided to make a house-to-house survey of the poor, and to classify them. Those who were 'undersettles', not being born in York, nor resident there for more than three years, were to be banished to where they came from. Those unable to work were to be given a greater allowance than before, at least a penny a day 'under which some poor creator cannot lyve' so that they need not beg. Those able to work were to be employed, while those rogues and 'strange beggars' unwilling to work were to be put in houses of correction for punishment until they agreed to work, or were banished. Stocks were erected in the city so that they could be punished in public. Only those with a licence from the corporation were permitted to beg, and even they were prohibited on all the church's great feast days 'both because it soundeth of popery, and also it is a breach of all good order'. Anyone who gave to beggars calling at his door was to be fined, part of the fine being awarded to the corporation's 'secret persons' specially appointed to report on their neighbours. Further fines were made on those who kept undersettles in their homes. This system was implemented by officers and overseers appointed for each ward, the records of the assessment collected from each householder and then distributed to the poor, being regularly checked by the Lord Mayor and Aldermen.[6]

Many of these provisions were confirmed in Parliament's Poor Laws of 1598 and 1601.[7] They required every parish to levy rates on property-owners to finance the relief of the impotent poor, with regular or occasional payments in cash or kind ('outdoor relief'), to set the able-bodied to work, and to bind pauper children to apprenticeships, so that they could learn skills to support themselves in adult life. Unrepentant rogues who refused to work were to be punished in houses of correction, while incapacitated paupers were to be housed in almshouses or poorhouses. Responsibility for the implementation of these Acts fell on an official called the Overseer of the Poor, who was to be chosen from among the churchwardens and other substantial householders in each parish. Throughout the following 240 years, all poor-law relief in England was based on this legislation.

In many parishes, particularly those in rural areas, outdoor relief was the major form of assistance given to the poor up to the late eighteenth century. It was relatively easy to leave families in their own homes, helping them by paying their rent, and providing them with a regular pension, and perhaps also clothing, footwear, and medical services.[8] Outdoor relief let the poor retain both their dignity and their personal freedom, but had the disadvantage of being relatively expensive, and it was unsuitable for the young, the old, the sick, and the mentally ill. The first workhouses, therefore, came into being in the urban centres, where these problems were more concentrated.

Up to the early eighteenth century an Act of Parliament was required before a workhouse could be established, which provides a further explanation why relatively few were set up, and why most paupers remained on outdoor relief.

However, Sheffield had a workhouse in 1630, Halifax in 1635, Leeds in 1638, Rotherham by 1660, Ripon in 1684, Wakefield in 1689, and Hull in 1698.[9] Of these, there were a number of failures. The Halifax workhouse was demolished in 1700, for example, while the Hull workhouse or 'Charity Hall' was converted into a Charity School, and the former outdoor relief or 'weekly pensions' continued.

The Early Eighteenth Century

By means of an Act of 1722 the overseers of the poor in every parish were enabled, with the consent of the vestry, to set up workhouses, to contract with persons or other parishes for lodging, keeping, and employing the poor, to take the profit of their work for the better maintenance of the poor, and to join with other parishes to implement these arrangements.[10] All who refused to go into the workhouse now forfeited their right to any form of alternative relief. Given these powers, many parishes opened new workhouses, or reformed the operation of their old ones. Beverley, Leeds, and Whitby implemented this Act in 1726, Hull in 1728, Sheffield in 1733, Barnsley in 1736, Knaresborough in 1737, and Bradford and Rothwell in 1738, along with numerous others. Its effectiveness may be judged by the experience of the parishioners in Beverley.[11] At a meeting held in the Town Hall in April 1726 they agreed to join several parishes together, to raise the local poor rate, and to appoint a committee to build a new workhouse capable of housing 100 inmates. When it opened in 1727, they

> gave notice to all the Poor, that the Weekly Allowances [outdoor relief] were to cease at *Midsummer*; that such as were not able to maintain themselves and Families, must apply to the Governors of the Workhouse, to be by Them Provided for. And tho' before the opening of the House, 116 received the Parish Allowance, not above 8 came in at first, and we have never exceeded 26 in the House all this (1728) winter, tho' all kinds of

Provisions have been excessively dear, and the Season
very sickly . . . I am persuaded if the House had not
been opened, the Overseers would not have had less
than 200 People upon their Hands.

Clearly very few were willing to give up their own homes
and their personal liberty unless they had absolutely no
alternative. As a result, most of the inmates were young
children and the elderly, neither of whom were able to work
effectively to help offset the cost of their keep, as originally
intended. Some with manual skills knitted, spun, undertook
sewing, or made lace, while the remainder unpicked old
ropes to form the oakum used for caulking ships' seams or
stopping up leaks. They might also undertake practical
work in the workhouse or its garden, or be hired out as
labourers, being allowed in that case to keep 2*d* out of every
shilling they earned, while the remainder was retained by
the Overseers.

In the larger of the workhouses the diet was carefully
regulated during the second quarter of the eighteenth
century, and was designed to provide foodstuffs similar in
character, quantity, and quality to those regularly consumed
by the local labouring population. Economy was essential,
however, in order to keep the poor rate as low as possible.
The following dietaries show the range of foods provided:

Leeds 1726[12]

	Breakfast	*Dinner*	*Supper*
Sun.	Bread and beer	Beef and broth	Milk porridge
Mon.	Beef broth	Rice milk	Milk porridge
Tues.	Milk porridge	Plumb puddings	Bread and beer
Wed.	Bread and cheese	Beef and broth	Milk porridge
Thurs.	Beef broth	Potatoes	Bread and cheese
Fri.	Bread and beer	Rice milk	Milk porridge
Sat.	Water porridge and treacle	Pease porridge	Bread and beer

11.
The Leeds workhouse was erected as a two-storey building in Lady Lane in 1638 (a). In 1740 it was extended to include a workroom, an infirmary, granary, brewhouse, washhouse, and coalhouse (b); while further extensions around 1806 enabled it to house the town's poor through to 1861 (c); when it was replaced by the new workhouse in Beckett Street (d). Drawing by P. Brears.

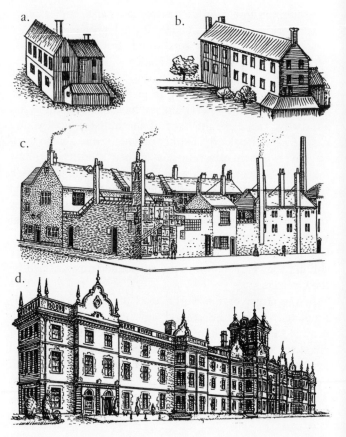

Beverley 1728[13]

As to their Diet, we allow Flesh Meat twice a Week, on other Days Rice-Milk, Hasty Puddings, Pease-Porridge, Baked Cakes, Puddings or Dumplings, for Breakfast and Supper, Bread and Milk in Summer, Milk Porridge in Winter and sometimes Bread and Cheese.

At Doncaster in 1747, inmates received each day 2 pints of milk porridge for breakfast, and bread and cheese and a mug of beer for supper. Their dinner on Sunday and Thursday was meat, roots, pudding, broth, bread and beer, and on other days they had pease-porridge or pudding or 'furmity' (frumenty), and beer in the afternoon.[14]

Rice milk (Leeds) was rice cooked to softness in water and then boiled up with milk, and frumenty was pearled wheat or barley treated in a similar manner, and probably enriched with currants.[15] The three dietaries show a remarkable uniformity, and include boiled meat twice a week as well as ample milk and cheese.

In the smaller workhouse dietaries appear to have been quite informal, the supply and preparation of food being very similar to that of any ordinary household. At Horbury, for example, the accounts for July 1747 show that a joint of meat, either beef, or leg or neck of mutton or a sheeps' heart, was purchased every week, along with either carrots or cabbage, a little salt, sugar, treacle and spices, and yeast for baking bread or oatcakes. The inmates also practised a degree of self-sufficiency by brewing their own beer from purchased supplies of malt, hops and yeast; by keeping a cow and processing its milk; and by maintaining an orchard. They even generated a modest income by selling their surplus produce, which included butter, pigeons, goose-berries, apples, and pig food in the form of the spent malt grains left after brewing.[16]

From this evidence it becomes immediately apparent that the inmates of the early eighteenth-century workhouses were well fed. Their diet compared very favourably with that of the local working community who were supporting them through the poor rate. The contemporary West Riding textile workers, for example, were having water-porridge for breakfast, occasional boiled meat and oatcake for midday dinner, and broth for supper. As Gamaliel Lloyd noted, salt beef, 'Water-Grewel & Onion & Bacon & Eggs, Oatcakes

and salt butter furnished the principal food of the People',
to support them throughout their fifteen-hour working day.[17]

The Late Eighteenth Century

The opening decades of the eighteenth century had seen a
considerable rise in the prosperity of the whole population
of England, with food prices becoming relatively low in
comparison to wages. In contrast, the latter half of the
century saw a complete reversal of this process. There was a
rapid rise in population, the wars with America and France
brought financial instability, the enclosure of thousands of
acres of common land robbed many small cottages of their
grazing rights, and the movement of people from the land
to the expanding industrial centres tended to leave old
people unsupported in rural areas. In addition a succession
of bad harvests between 1764 and 1775 caused the price of
corn, and hence of most other foodstuffs, to soar.[18]

In these circumstances it is not surprising that the number
of paupers began to grow, thus increasing the financial and
administrative burden on their parishes. Parliament res-
ponded in 1782 by passing Gilbert's Act, which encouraged
parishes to join together in order to manage the care of the
poor more effectively. The advantages of this arrangement
had already been proved in York, where seventeen city
parishes had closed down their individual workhouses in
1767 in order to set up a unified establishment for 150
paupers in a former cotton factory in Marygate.[19] As a
result of Gilbert's Act a number of new workhouses were
built in the county, the North Riding's thirty-five workhouses of 1776 rising to seventy-three in 1803, and eighty-
five in 1815.[20] In the West Riding, meanwhile, the ninety-
nine workhouses of 1776 had risen to 151 in 1803.[21]

In spite of these improved facilities, the cost of maintaining
the poor still placed a considerable burden on those who
paid the ever-increasing poor rates. 'The principle of the
poor's law is to impose a tax on the industrious, to be paid to
the profligate', wrote Robert Brown in 1799, 'but we grant
at once that those who from age, disease or dibility, are

unable to provide for themselves, ought to be furnished with the means of subsistance by the community with which they are connected.'[22] A contemporary Yorkshire farmer also recorded that in his village the poor were treated with the utmost kindness and humanity, and hence had become more expensive to maintain than ever before, since 'the more bountiful we are, the more heedless and extravagent [sic] they are, I speak of the haughty and insolent; the aged and helpless will, I trust, ever meet with tenderness and compassionate assistance from their fellow creatures.'[23] The quality of this 'compassionate assistance' is clearly seen from the following account of workhouse dietaries of the 1790s, especially when they are compared with the localised circumstances experienced by the ordinary working population within the county.[24]

In late eighteenth-century Yorkshire, oatmeal was still one of the most widely-used foodstuffs, virtually every workhouse serving porridge made with either milk or water for breakfast each day, accompanied by either milk, boiled milk, broth, beer, or bread. In many workhouses, including Headingley, Southowram, and Stokesley, porridge and its various accompaniments appeared every day at suppertime, too, while in many others it was replaced by broth and bread on a number of evenings. In both Leeds and Ecclesfield,[25] porridge formed five suppers each week and broth the remaining two; in Hull porridge formed two suppers, broth a further two, and bread and cheese the remaining three, while in Sheffield porridge formed only one supper, the others alternating between broth or beer, both eaten with bread. In those workhouses where no porridge was served at supper, its place was taken by bread; Pocklington serving bread and milk every evening, for example, while Ovenden served bread accompanied by either milk, butter, or cheese. In those areas where oatcake was generally used by the working population, it formed part of the workhouse diet, the Eccleshill dietary specifically stating that its 'bread' was usually oatcake, but sometimes wheaten bread.

The greatest variety of workhouse food appeared at the midday dinner, the main meal of the day. Most workhouses provided two meat dinners each week, usually on Sundays and either Wednesdays or Thursdays, although at Leeds meat appeared on Sundays only, while at a few others (such as Sheffield and Ovenden), it appeared on Sundays, Tuesdays, and Thursdays. For reasons of economy, to render the cheaper cuts of meat more tender, and to provide a ready supply of nourishing broth, the joints of beef or mutton were usually boiled, and served with a selection of potatoes, vegetables, bread, dumplings, suet puddings, and beer. Throughout the remainder of the week the dinners were composed of the cheapest and most filling foods, such as puddings and sauce, dumplings, frumenty (pearled wheat or barley porridge), rice milk, bread and butter, bread and cheese, or pea soup. Usually a different dish from this selection appeared each day of the week, but in some workhouses, including Halifax and Southowram, a mono- tonous diet of potatoes, butter, milk, and bread or oatcake was served on the five non-meat days.

Regarding the size of the individual portions, the dietaries from Hull, Leeds, and Headingley suggest that men usually received some 8 oz. of meat, 7 oz. of bread, 4 oz. of cheese, 11 oz. of flour in cakes or dumplings, and 8 oz. of rice and 5 oz. of sugar in rice milk whenever these foods were served. Women and children of different ages received proportionally less.

Where the dietaries note the quantity and quality of food eaten by working people outside the workhouse, it is noticeable that their food was generally comparable with that provided for the inmates. In Stokesley, for example, the local diet of bread, milk and tea, potatoes and a little meat was virtually identical to that served in the workhouse, while at Ecclesfield the local poverty diet of onion porridge and boiled nettles made the food provided in the workhouse appear positively luxurious. In general terms, the poor in the north of England were much better fed than were their contemporaries in the south, largely due to their economic methods of cookery, and their reliance on well-established traditional foods such as hasty pudding, crowdy, frumenty, and pease-pottage, together with the newly adopted potatoes and rice, as described by Sir Frederick Eden.[26]

At many workhouses traditional festive foods were also provided at the appropriate times of the year – Leeds serving roast beef and a pound of spice cake at Christmas; and veal and bacon at Easter and Whitsuntide, with further spice cakes. Sheffield, too, provided similar fare, but with plum puddings replacing the cakes.[27] At Knaresborough special treats were occasionally provided, the Master promising the inmates that 'if they would get their work done they should all go to Harrogate Races and I would go with them and by them every one sum ginsbread . . . I told them they mud all be good and carefull and not waste all their brass on halfpenny cakes and peny cakes.'[28] Richer foods also played their part in the sick-room, as may be seen from the following extracts from various workhouse account books of this period:[29]

1777	'By sugar for the children in small pox'
1779	'Tea and sugar for women lying in'
1808	'Brandy for the cow'
1791	'I went into Chamber and got her a cupful of raisin wine and she drunk it and came about bravely that day and did her work'.
1792	'She was but poorly but my wife got her sum tea and gruel'

Some impression of the ways in which the dining rooms were used and the food was served may be obtained from a variety of sources. The well-organised Leeds workhouse printed its rules and orders, and instructed the Master to read them out in the dining room at dinnertime once every month. They include:

19.   That the Dishes be washed twice a Day or
        oftner by the Cooks, and the Dining-room
        Tables be washed every Day.

23.   That Prayers be read in the public Dining-
        Room every Morning before Breakfast, and
        every evening before Supper; and that Grace
        be duly said at Dinner and Supper.

24.   That all the Poor in this house who are able
        to attend Prayers, sit decently at their Meals,
        avoid talking, and make no attempt to go out
        of the Dining Room till Thanks are returned,
        and in Default in any of these Particulars, to
        lose their next Meal.

29.   [None] of the Poor maintained in this House
        shall carry any Bread, Cheese or other
        Provisions without Leave of the Master out
        of the common Dining-Room.

31.   . . . to prevent Disputes which may arise
        from telling Lies, the Offender shall, by
        Order of the Master, be set to stand upon a
        Stool in the Dining-Room during Dinner-
        Time with a Paper fixed on his or her Breast,
        whereon shall be written *Infamous Liar*, and
        shall also lose that meal.

In addition, every person was to find his own knife and
fork.[30] By implementing these rules with a humane
disposition and firm, even temper, the Master, Mr Linsley,
became beloved, respected, and obeyed with cheerfulness,
and so enabled the poor under his care to live in perfect
harmony with each other.[31] This was an extremely rare
occurrence. The same order did not prevail elsewhere. In
Sheffield, for example, the inmates carried their breakfasts
and suppers of porridge and bread up the narrow and steep
stairs to their 9 ft 6 in. square bedrooms, where they could
sit on one of the beds they shared with up to three others.
Here dinners were taken in the hall, the old people dining

first, leaving the food they did not eat on the table to form part of the dinner of the children who followed them.[32] In the smaller workhouses, the circumstances could be even more squalid, one man remembering a scene in Pudsey workhouse with 'large black bowls filled with oatmeal porridge and milk, and a big podgy person who figures as Master filling black earthenware mugs with a ladle, and the poor miserably clad people hobbling away with their meal to their room, which was not very tidy or overclean'.[33] The 'black earthenware mugs' were undoubtedly the local 'meas-pots', round-bodied vessels from which a pint of porridge, broth, or other food could be spooned without the need to sit at table.

Clearly, the standards of care varied from one workhouse to another throughout the county, but the overall picture is one of a society generally succeeding in caring for those unable to support themselves, and usually feeding them better than many ordinary people who were in full employment could feed themselves. To do this at a time of rising prices and great social change represents no small achievement.

The Early Nineteenth Century

In 1836 a detailed inventory was taken of the contents of the small township workhouse at Ovenden, just north of Halifax.[34] This makes it possible to build an accurate picture of pauper life during this period. The house was provisioned as if it were expecting to withstand a long siege. In the kitchen chamber there were 26 stones of bacon, 48 lb of hogs lard, and 5 stones of beef, along with large chests, cupboards and sacks holding four loads of potatoes, a pack and a half of flour, a pack of oatmeal, and three strikes of malt, and the beam-scales and weights required for weighing them out. The cellar and pantry housed the community's six barrels of beer, the kneading kit, baking board and rolling pin used when baking, and the basting spoon and 'haster' (or Dutch oven) for roasting the meat. These rooms also served as a dairy, where the six cow-buckets of milk from their seven cows were strained through two 'siles' and left to settle in three lead and four pottery milk bowls overnight until the cream could be lifted off with the skimmer into five cream pots. Once sufficient cream had been accumulated, it was poured into the churn, and agitated until it turned to butter. The buttermilk having been poured off, the butter was clashed [beaten] in the wooden butter bowl to remove the surplus liquid and beat in salt from the salt bowl. When it had been weighed on the butter-scales, and impressed with the carved wooden print, it was placed in one of the three butter baskets ready either for use or for sale. The mouse trap and rat trap would, it was hoped, prevent hungry rodents from nibbling this dairy produce.

A set-pot or copper in the back kitchen provided the hot water both for washing clothes in the washing machine, and for brewing the workhouse's beer in two brewing tubs. The two bakestones here were presumably used for baking oatcakes when Hannah Snowden came in to do her regular four-day baking sessions. When removed from the bake-stones, the oatcakes would be hung from the bread creel overhead, where they would soon dry out.

The kitchen itself was equipped with a range comprising an oven, a pan, an iron fireback, and a screen, together with all the brigs [supporting frames], grid iron, frying pan, iron kettle, dripping pans, coal skip, and fire irons necessary for cooking. Here, too, were the five candlesticks and three oil lamps used to light the house, the brushes for cleaning and whitewashing it, and the warming pan for airing the beds on cold nights. Rather more ominous were the thumbscrews and four leg irons apparently necessary for restraining some of the inmates.

The housebody or living-room was a large appartment pleasantly furnished with an oak chest, oak clock, oak drawers and cupboard, a desk and a stool, a longsettle, four tables, eight chairs, six forms, and two turnup beds which folded up against the wall when not in use. This was where the paupers dined, their pottage being cooked in three large pans, and the water for their tea and coffee boiled in a copper kettle heated over either of this room's two fireplaces. These and the other foods were served out in forty small cans accompanied by forty spoons and cutlery from the kitchen. Presumably the paupers spent their evenings together here, too, enjoying the tobacco, twist, snuff, and apples bought in for them by the Overseer.

During the daytime the able-bodied paupers made woollen cloth using the spinning wheels, swift [machine for reeling thread], and three looms standing in their main bedroom or 'Great Chamber', carried out domestic work in the workhouse, or helped to operate a well-equipped home farm. The Ovenden workhouse also ran a quarry, where the paupers used blasting and stone-cutting tools to make the sets and kerbs required for road-building. In almost every way the local paupers would have found the communal life here very similar indeed to that which they had experienced in their own cottages and farmsteads, but this intimate domestic scale of indoor relief was soon to come to an end.

In the period of political and social unrest following the Napoleonic Wars, attitudes to the poor hardened. Against a background of rising expenditure on maintaining the poor and an ever increasing number of paupers, many people began to believe that supporting the poor at anything above the most basic subsistence level positively encouraged idleness and vice. The Rev. George Young of Whitby had no doubts about the situation. In the half century between 1760 and 1810 the cost of relieving the poor in this north-eastern port had risen eightfold, from £311 to £2,467, while the number of paupers in the workhouse had more than tripled, from 35 to 128. 'Perhaps there are few places where the poor are better provided for than in Whitby', he wrote:[35]

A poor-house, as now conducted, is often a receptacle for vice, rather than an asylum for honest poverty. The door is open, indeed, for the industrious poor;

but it admits with equal facility characters the most abandoned and worthless, with whom the virtuous abhor to associate. The most numerous tenants of the poor-house too often consists of such as have reduced themselves to poverty by idleness and drunkenness; lewd girls, with their illegitimate off-spring and others who are the very dregs of society. What is the consequence? The many hundreds that are levied on industrious tradesmen and worthy citizens, are chiefly expended in supporting the lazy and profligate, while the real objects of charity pine away in private, and bear up almost to the last extremity, under the pressure of old age, affliction and distress, rather than herd with wretches so depraved.

Similar views continued to be expressed throughout the country, so that the government appointed the Poor Law Commission in 1832 'to make diligent and full inquiry into the practical operation of the laws for the relief of the poor in England and Wales, and into the manner in which those laws were administered, and to report their opinion as to what beneficial alterations could be made'.[36] Among the questions they circulated, the Commissioners asked if a family could subsist on its earnings, and, if so, on what food? One North Riding respondent stated that a labourer and his family could subsist on bread or oatmeal, potatoes, milk and bacon, with meat once or twice a week.[37] This was less than many contemporary workhouse diets, as may be seen in the following typical local examples:

Hedon [38]

	Breakfast	*Dinner*	*Supper*
Sun.	Milk & 6 oz. bread	Beef & potato pie	Milk & 6 oz. bread
Mon.	Milk & 6 oz. bread	Pea soup or broth & 6 oz. bread	Milk & 6 oz. bread

Tues.	Milk & 6 oz. bread	Suet pudding	Milk & 6 oz. bread
Wed.	Milk & 6 oz. bread	Broth, 6 oz. of beef 4 oz. bread, & a portion of potatoes	Broth & 6 oz. bread
Thurs.	Milk & 6 oz. bread	Rice milk & 4 oz. bread	Milk & 6 oz. bread
Fri.	Milk & 6 oz. bread	Broth 6 oz. beef, 4 oz. bread, & a portion of potatoes	Broth & 6 oz. bread
Sat.	Milk & 6 oz. bread	Frumenty & 4 oz. bread	Milk & 6 oz. bread

Women to have tea for breakfast and supper instead of milk.

Leeds[39]

	Breakfast	*Dinner*	*Supper*
Sun.	Milk porridge	6 oz. boiled mutton or beef etc. 6 oz. bread with potatoes	Milk porridge
Mon.	Milk porridge	Broth from Sunday's meat well seasoned, mixed with vegetables 6 oz. bread	Milk porridge
Tues.	Milk porridge	As Sunday	Milk porridge
Wed.	Milk porridge	As Monday	Milk porridge
Thurs.	Milk porridge	As Sunday	Milk porridge
Fri.	Milk porridge	As Monday	Milk porridge
Sat.	Milk porridge	4 oz. dumplings with 1 tablespoon treacle, 6 oz. bread, and 2 oz. cheese	Milk porridge

Each adult to have 1 pt beer every day.

The Commissioners noted similar circumstances in other parts of England.[40] In Reading the Governor gave the paupers 'a bellyful. We never stint them. I stand by the children myself and see they have a bellyful three times a day . . . Good wholesome victuals . . . We give them meat three times a week . . . We never weigh anything, and there is no stint.' In Oxford the paupers were 'better fed than they could expect to be in their own homes. The house is not an object of terror, but rather of desire to the young and able bodied . . .'; while in Kidderminster they were 'in a better situation than the independent poor [and] they disposed of portions of their food, in order to spend money at the ale-house'. The same routine was followed at Scarborough, where the inmates pooled their bread ration in order to sell it off to raise money for snuff and tea.[41] From evidence such as this, the Commissioners were forced to conclude that[42]

> In-doors Relief, that which is given, within the walls
> of the Poor-House, or as it is usually, but very seldom
> properly denominated, the Workhouse, is also subject
> to great mal-administration. . . . in the absence of
> classification, discipline and employment, and the
> extravagance of allowance. . . .

The food was good; in fact it was generally better both in variety and in amount than that consumed not only by the labourers, but by most of the householders who actually paid the poor rate.

To remedy this situation, Parliament passed the Poor Law Amendment Act, better known as the New Poor Law, in 1834. Its aim was to keep paupers out of the workhouse by making life within comparatively unpleasant by means of a strictly enforced discipline. Instead of keeping the paupers in small parish workhouses, controlled entirely by leading members of the local community, they were now to be gathered together in large union workhouses serving a number of parishes, and controlled by locally elected guardians who were bound to implement the directions, orders, and regulations of a central body of Poor Law Commissioners for England and Wales. This legislation was not popular. The local gentry strongly objected to the removal of their former power, patronage, and other indirect advantages, greatly resenting the interference of a powerful outside body in the affairs of their own locality. The poor, both inside and outside the workhouse, had even more reason to complain. They had lost the right to outdoor relief, unless they could obtain the consent of two justices; the new workhouses were large, impersonal institutions lacking any of the comfortable, relaxed family atmosphere of many of their smaller predecessors; and married couples and families were split up and kept permanently in separate wards – an inhuman practice in direct contradiction to God's law.

In rural areas, such as the East Riding, ten new poor law unions were formed in 1835–7, but in the industrial areas, particularly in the West Riding, the legislation met with the strongest possible opposition. Powerful and wily leaders such as Richard Oastler and John Fielden used a variety of tactics which effectively meant that Parliament was unable to implement its plans here for some years, and even when it did so (as with the establishment of the Bradford Union in 1837), it often led to riots.[43] The Todmorden Union set up in 1875 was the last to succumb, after which all poor relief in the county operated under the 1834 Act.[44]

The harsh conditions within the reformed workhouses earned them a reputation for oppression and inhumanity. G. R. Wyther Baxter described them in his book *The Book of the Bastilles*, entitled after the great French fortress, prison, and symbol of tyranny which was stormed and demolished by the revolutionary mob in 1789.[45] Contemporary newspapers immediately adopted this description. For example Oastler wrote in the *Northern Star* of 10 March 1838: 'The real object of [the New Poor Law] is to lower wages and punish poverty as a crime. Remember also that children and parents are lying frequently in the same Bastille without seeing one another, or knowing one another's fate.' Just as a term in prison became associated with porridge, so life within the workhouse became associated with the universal gruel, or broth, now christened 'Bastille Soup'. Professor Moorman's poem on working life in Yorkshire, 'The Dalesman's Litany', uses this term to describe a typical scene in one of our greatest Victorian cities:[46]

I've seen grey fog creep ower Leeds Brig
As thick as bastile soup;
I've lived wheer fowks were stowed away
Like rabbits in a coop.
I've watched snow float down Bradforth Beck
As black as ebiny;
Frae Hunslet, Holbeck, Wibsey Slack,
Gooid Lord, deliver me!

In practical terms, the new union workhouses were
admirably designed to house and feed efficiently their neatly
segregated communities of infants, boys, girls, men, women,
the mentally or physically infirm, and vagrants. Behind
their brick and stone façades, perhaps built in the fashionable
yet economic 'Jacobethan' style, lay the capacious wards,
kitchens, dining rooms, wash-houses, etc., all equipped with
robust and practical furniture and utensils. As a visitor to
the Doncaster workhouse noted in 1864, after

> passing through the kitchen, with its immense fire-
> range and cooking apparatus, the larder was reached.
> Piles of bread loaves, pancheons of milk, legs and
> shoulders of mutton, and a troughful of pickled beef,
> dispelled all notions of scarcity; . . . We had seen
> nothing yet of actual misery, we scarcely observed a
> face in which there was a lurking discontent. The
> food, though not luxurious, or improvidently
> distributed, must be abundant for we beheld nothing
> but health. We know that health is dependent upon
> cleanliness, ventilation, and sufficient food, . . . and
> the food must be ample for the purposes of health,
> otherwise there would be sickness.[47]

The way in which the new dietaries were decided and
enforced is clearly illustrated from the records of the Carlton
workhouse near Otley. Until 1864 it had been a Gilbert
Union institution, after which it joined the Wharfedale

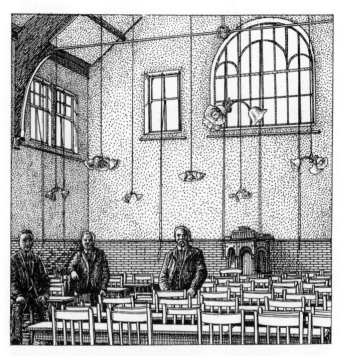

12.
The dining room, Pontefract Union workhouse, *c.* 1900. Note the narrow tables, with chairs ranged along one side only, so that the inmates had little chance of conversation, and had their attention directed to the reading desk. Drawing by P. Brears.

Union, the diet being revised to meet the requirements of the new regime. In September 1869 the existing diet was submitted by the local Guardians of the Poor to the national Poor Law Board:[48]

	Breakfast	*Dinner*	*Supper*
Sun.	Bread & coffee	Boiled beef & peas, beer	Boiled milk & bread
Mon.	Oatmeal porridge & milk	Broth & suet dumplings	Flour porridge, milk & treacle
Tues.	Oatmeal porridge & milk	Meat & potato pie, beer	Tea & bread
Wed.	Oatmeal porridge & milk	Broth & rice pudding	Boiled milk & bread
Thurs.	Oatmeal porridge & milk	Beef & potatoes with veg. from the garden, beer	Boiled milk & bread
Fri.	Oatmeal porridge & milk	Broth & dumplings	Boiled milk & bread

13.
Tea in the children's section of Pontefract workhouse *c*. 1900. Here a distinctly domestic atmosphere was achieved by putting flowers on the table and the mantelpiece. Matron is about to fill the large mugs with tea from the urn placed before her. Drawing by P. Brears.

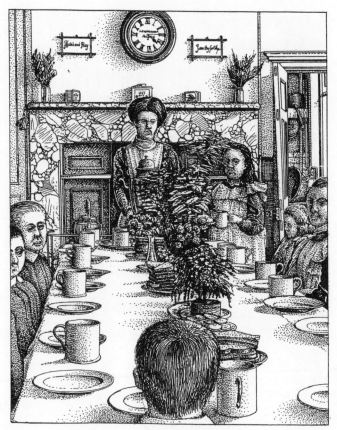

The Board suggested a number of alterations: milk porridge to replace the tea on Tuesdays; the quantity of pudding served for dinner on Thursdays should be increased from 12 oz. to 14 oz. for adults; while the children should have 2 oz. of bread for Thursday dinners, and 1 oz. of rice pudding on Fridays. The Board then went on to state that it was 'unusual and unnecessary to allow beer, and also undesirable to allow tea for the aged'. At first the Guardians stood their ground and refused to strike out the beer, but

eventually they had to accept this miserable demand, beer
being provided only on the authority of the medical officer
when it was necessary for the health of a pauper.

Once the Poor Law Board had agreed the dietary table,
they issued a printed order to the Guardians of the Poor of
the union, which stated that

1. The Paupers described in the following Tables,
   who may be received and maintained in the
   Workhouse of the Wharfedale Union in the
   County of York, shall, during their residence
   therein, be dieted and maintained with food and
   in the manner described as follows; that is to say:

	Breakfast	*Dinner*	*Supper*
Sun.	7 oz. bread, 1½ pts porridge	5 oz. cooked meat, 10 oz. potatoes or other vegetables, 2 oz. bread	1 pt tea with ½ oz. sugar, 8 oz. bread
Mon.	7 oz. bread, 1½ pts porridge	1½ pt broth & 6 oz. bread	1 pt rice milk, 7 oz. bread
Tues.	7 oz. bread, 1½ pts porridge	16 oz. suet pudding with treacle sauce	1 pt porridge, 7 oz. bread
Wed.	7 oz. bread, 1½ pts porridge	As Sunday	As Monday
Thurs.	7 oz. bread, 1½ pts porridge	As Monday	As Tuesday
Fri.	7 oz. bread, 1½ pts porridge	As Sunday	As Tuesday
Sat.	7 oz. bread, 1½ pts porridge	8 oz. rice pudding with treacle, 4 oz. bread, and 2 oz. cheese	As Monday

[This was the diet for the able-bodied men; the same
diet was provided for able-bodied women, for aged
and infirm male and female imbeciles, and for
children between 2 and 5, 5 and 9, and 9 and 16, but
with lesser quantities appropriate to their
requirements.]

141

2. Youths of either sex above 16 years of age, resident in the said Workhouse, shall be dieted as able-bodied men and women respectively, and infants under the age of 2 years and sick persons, shall be dieted in such manner as the Medical Officer for the Workhouse shall direct.

3. The Master of the said Workhouse shall cause two or more copies of so much of this Order as comprises the above Tables, legibly written or printed in large type, to be hung up in the most public places of such Workhouse, and renewed from time to time, so that such copies may always be kept fair and legible.

4. Provided, that nothing herein contained shall be taken to rescind or alter any regulation of the Poor Law Board contained in their Order, bearing the date Seventh day of March One thousand eight hundred and sixty-one, addressed to the Guardians of the Poor of the Wharfedale Union, which applies to the subject of the diet of the Paupers at the Workhouse of the said Union.

5. Provided also, that on the occasion of any public Festival or Thanksgiving, the Guardians may depart from the Regulations herein contained, in such manner as they shall think fit.

Given under our Hand and Seal of Office, this Thirtieth day of October 1869
George Gosehem, President
Arthur W. Peel, Secretary.

Recipes to be used;
1. *Soup* Per gallon of water.
        24 oz. beef (to remain in the soup) 14 oz. split peas, 4 oz. oatmeal, 16 oz. potatoes, 8 oz. bones, 3 oz. carrots

2. *Broth*   Per gallon of meat liquor in which the
             meat was boiled, 4 oz. oatmeal, parsley,
             pepper, salt.
3. *Suet Pudding*
             7 oz. flour, 1½ oz. suet, 2 oz. skimmed
             milk, water & salt
4. *Rice Pudding*
             3 oz. rice, ½ oz. suet, ½ oz. sugar, ½ pt
             skimmed milk, salt, spice & water.

The precision of this diet is typical of those accepted by
the Poor Law Board, as may be seen by the following
example:

Leeds 1897[49]

	Breakfast	*Dinner*	*Supper*
Sun.	6 oz. bread, 1 pt cocoa, ½ oz. butter	4 oz. cooked meat, 10 oz. potatoes and vegetables, 3 oz. bread	7 oz. bread 1 pt tea ½ oz. butter
Mon.	6 oz. bread, 1 pt coffee, ½ oz. butter	1 pt soup, 6 oz. bread	7 oz. bread, 1 pt tea ½ oz. butter
Tues.	As Sunday	14 oz. meat and potato pie	7 oz. bread, 1 pt tea ½ oz. butter
Wed.	As Monday	As Sunday	7 oz. bread 1 pt tea ½ oz. butter
Thurs.	As Sunday	As Monday	7 oz. bread 1 pt tea ½ oz. butter
Fri.	As Monday	As Sunday	7 oz. bread 1 pt tea ½ oz. butter
Sat.	As Monday	14 oz. Irish stew, 4 oz. bread	7 oz. bread 1 pt tea ½ oz. butter

CHILDREN

		2-6	6-9	9-12	12-16 years
	Breakfast				
	Bread	3 oz.	4 oz.	5 oz.	6 oz.
	Milk & water		¾ pt	¾ pt	¾ pt
	Pure milk	½ pt			
	Cocoa (on Sunday)	½ pt	¾ pt	¾ pt	¾ pt
	10 a.m.	2 oz. bread for each child			
	Dinner				
Sun.	Cooked meat	2 oz.	3 oz.	3½ oz.	4 oz.
	Potatoes & veg.	4 oz.	6 oz.	8 oz.	8 oz.
	Bread	2 oz.	3 oz.	3 oz.	3 oz.
Mon.	Soup	½ pt	¾ pt	¾ pt	1 pt
	Bread	3 oz.	4 oz.	6 oz.	6 oz.
Tues.	Meat & potato pie	6 oz.	8 oz.	10 oz.	12 oz.
	Bread	2 oz.	3 oz.	3 oz.	3 oz.
Wed. Thurs.	As Sunday Currant pudding	6 oz.	8 oz.	10 oz.	12 oz.
Fri. Sat.	As Sunday Rice with treacle sauce	6 oz.	8 oz.	10 oz.	2 oz.
	Supper				
Sun.	Bread	5 oz.	6 oz.	7 oz.	8 oz.
	Milk & water		¾ pt	¾ pt	¾ pt
	Pure milk	½ pt			
	Treacle	¼ oz.	½ oz.	½ oz.	¾ oz.
Mon.	Water porridge	¼ pt	½ pt	¾ pt	1 pt
	Pure milk	½ pt	½ pt	½ pt	½ pt
Tues. Thurs. Sat.	As Sunday				
Wed. Fri.	As Monday				

In 1897 the President of the Local Government Board, which now directed national policies for operating workhouses, appointed a Committee of Enquiry to gather information on the effectiveness of their existing diets. As a result, new regulations came into force throughout England and Wales on 25 March 1901.[50] Alternative rations were specified for each meal, and Boards of Guardians were at liberty to make a selection from these when planning their diets. They had to ensure, however, that no fewer than two boiled or roast meat dinners (beef, mutton, or pork in suitable rotation) were provided weekly, and, with the exception of those meals, that no two dinners were alike during one week. The paupers were given no alternative but to accept the new arrangements, as is clearly seen in the following extract from the *Manchester Guardian* of 29 March 1901:

> At the Bradford Workhouse yesterday the new dietary table of the Local Government Board came into operation. When served with gruel instead of tea, according to the order, the women rose in a body and left the room. Three women who were ringleaders were yesterday brought before the Stipendary Magistrate. These women, with others, had refused to work on the food, and had also behaved in a rowdy manner to the Workhouse Master. The Master said the gruel consisted of three ounces of oatmeal, a pint of water, half an ounce of treacle, and salt to taste. Each defendant was sent to prison for a week.

The fact that complaints about the standard and quality of the food could result in a prison sentence was presumably effective in ensuring that all the paupers appeared well satisfied. However, the opening years of the twentieth century saw a radical change in attitude to the relief of the poor, particularly as the Liberal Party, spurred on by the emerging Labour Party, began to seek reforms at both local and national levels. In 1909, for example, Benjamin North, Guardian of the Poor and Labour Member on the Distress Committee for Crosland Moor near Huddersfield, began to expose the totally unacceptable practices of his local workhouse.[51] Here, he stated, the quantity of fat mixed into the rice milk made many of the aged inmates quite ill, the alternative diet recommended by the medical officer being totally ignored. How could this be when the Master served the Guardians with sumptuous 2s or half-crown teas for which they paid only 6d each? And why did the Master keep 300 hens consuming £10 12s 6d in corn every six months, and only record twenty hens in his books?

At the same time, the Government began to introduce legislation which would eventually see the final closure of the workhouses and their replacement by the supportive services of a modern welfare state. In 1906 local authorities were permitted to provide free school meals to poor children, so that they would be able to take advantage of their years of compulsory education, while in 1908 a non-contributory pension of 5s a week was made available to all poor people over 70 years old. This was followed in 1911 by the start of National Insurance, to provide relief in times of sickness or unemployment. The well-deserved popular support for the new pensions in Yorkshire was beautifully expressed in F. W. Moorman's poem 'Lord George' [i.e. Lloyd George]:[52]

> I'd walk frae here to Skipton,
> Ten mile o' clarty [muddy] lanes,
> If I might see him face to face
> An' thank him for his pains.
> He's ta'en me out o't Bastile
> He's gi'en me life that's free
> Five shillin a week for cheating Death
> Is what Lord George gives me.

He gives me leet an' firin'.
An' flour to bake i't' yoon. [oven]
I've tea to mash for ivery meal
An sup all t' afternoon . . . .
I know a vast o' widdows
That's seen their seventieth year
Lord George he addles brass [earns money] for all
Though lots on't goes for beer

The workhouse system eventually came to an end shortly after the Second World War, when the Boards of Guardians were dissolved, and many of the union workhouses were converted into general or geriatric hospitals. No one was sad to see them go. Over the centuries they had acquired an evil reputation, and it was certainly true that they had witnessed scenes of great brutality and degradation when subject to the whims of overbearing masters and ineffectual administrations. Be that as it may, it is well to remember that the living conditions and food they provided were almost always a great improvement on those available to the poorest sections of society fighting for survival in the squalid world outside. Throughout this period generations of impoverished inhabitants of both rural hovels and over-crowded town-centre tenements had to suffer the privations of disease, bad housing, polluted air, water, and surroundings, and a diet with little or no variety at the most basic subsistence level. They rarely saw meat, and could spend years on a nutritionally deprived diet of a little porridge and even less bacon, small amounts of tea or coffee, and white bread alone in addition. In comparison, the workhouses provided a good diet which undoubtedly saved the lives of hundreds of thousands of people who would otherwise have starved on the streets.

The real fear of the workhouse came from the loss of personal freedom and family relationships experienced on entering its stark, impersonal, and prison-like regime. There was further degradation in having to admit that you were such a miserable failure that you had to give up all your personal liberties and place the control of your life into the hands of others. It is not surprising that the fear of entering the workhouse, however disguised under a new name, still evokes a strong reaction in many elderly people even today. In 1963, when Joan Richards worked at Headlands Hospital, the former Pontefract workhouse, she found that many old people still dreaded the thought of entering the workhouse:[53]

> They never call it Headlands, or Northgate Lodge. When one old man was admitted his family agreed 'Whatever you do, don't tell him he's in Headlands.' He was doing fine, and he really liked the place until one day someone forgot. 'It is nice in here isn't it? I never thought Headlands would be as nice as this.' After that he went down rapidly. As soon as ever he realised where he was he couldn't cope. He still thought of it as the workhouse. It takes a lot longer to change attitudes than it does names.

Notes and References

1. J. Ashton, *Modern Street Ballads* (London, 1888), p. 351.
2. Sir Hugh Cholmley, *The Memoirs of Sir Hugh Chomley* (London, 1787), p. 56.
3. 12 Richard II, 11 c. 7 (1388); 11 Henry VII, c. 2 (1495); 19 Henry VIII, c. 12 (1504); 22 Henry VIII, c. 12 (1531); and 27 Henry VIII, c. 25 (1536).
4. 1 Edward VI, c. 3 (1547) repealed 3 & 4 Edward VI, c. 16 (1550).
5. 5 & 6 Edward VI, c. 2 (1551); 2 & 3 Philip & Mary, c. 5 (1555); 5 Elizabeth I, c. 3 (1563); and 14 Elizabeth I, c. 5 (1572).
6. A. Raine (ed.), *York Civic Records, vol. 8* (Yorkshire Records Series, 119, 1952), p. 157, also pp. 35, 47, 54, 96, 118, 133, 141.
7. 39 Elizabeth I, c. 3 (1598) and 43 Elizabeth I, c. 2 (1601).
8. For example, see the Carleton-in-Craven Overseers Accounts. Leeds Reference Library M1C/352. 04274/c765.
9. K. Grady, *The Georgian Public Buildings of Leeds and the West Riding* (Thoresby Society Publications, 62, no. 133, 1987), pp. 173, 157, 161, 172, 171, 179.
10. 9 George I, c. 7.
11. *An Account of the Work-Houses in Great Britain in the Year 1732* (London, 1786), pp. 169–74.
12. The Leeds Workhouse Committee Order Book, Leeds City Archives LO/MI.

13. *An Account of the Work-Houses . . . 1732*, p. 174.
14. C. W. Hatfield, *Historical Notices of Doncaster* (Doncaster 1866), p. 287.
15. For recipes for pease porridge, rice-milk, and furmity, see H. Glasse, *The Art of Cookery* (London, 1747), p. 79, and for hasty pudding, p. 80. The workhouse versions probably omitted some of the sweetening and spices.
16. K. Bartlett, *Horbury Workhouse 1747–1789* (Horbury, 1988), p. 3.
17. P. Brears, *Traditional Food in Yorkshire* (Edinburgh, 1987), pp. 6–9.
18. J. C. Drummond and A. Wilbraham, *The Englishman's Food*, revised by D. F. Hollingsworth (London, 1957), pp. 171–3.
19. C. B. Knight, *A History of the City of York* (York, 1944), pp. 540, 583.
20. R. P. Hastings, *Poverty and the Poor Law in the North Riding of Yorkshire c.1780–1837* (Borthwick Papers, 61, 1982), pp. 21–3.
21. *Abstract of . . . An Act for Procuring Returns Relative to the Maintenance of the Poor in England* [43 George III 1803] (1804), p. 656.
22. R. Brown, *General View of the Agriculture of the West Riding of Yorkshire* (Edinburgh, 1799), pp. 25–6.
23. Ibid., p. 29.
24. See Sir Frederick Eden, *The State of the Poor (1797)* abridged and ed. A. G. L. Rogers (London, 1928), for all the dietaries discussed in this section except for 25 below.
25. G. E. Fussell, *The English Rural Labourer* (London, 1949), p. 85.
26. Eden, p. 101.
27. Ibid., pp. 360, 363.
28. Master's Day Book for Knaresborough Workhouse, 1788–92, Yorkshire Archaeological Society, MS 439, and quoted in M. Slack, *Yorkshire Fare* (Clapham, Yorks., 1979), p. 8.
29. Slack, p. 8.
30. *Rules and Orders for Relieving and Employing the Poor of the Township of Leeds* (Leeds, 1771).
31. Eden, p. 361.
32. Ibid., p. 363.
33. B. Strong, 'Pudsey Workhouse', *Old West Riding* 2 (1982), p. 32.
34. Calderdale Archives, HAS 211.
35. G. Young, *A History of Whitby* (Whitby, 1817), pp. 593, 598, 599.
36. Quoted in *Encyclopaedia Britannica*, vol. 22 (Cambridge, 1911), p. 74.
37. Hastings, p. 25.
38. Humberside County Record Office, Beverley, MS DDHE 17/33, quoted in Slack, p. 11.
39. *Appendix to 1st Report from the Commissioners on the Poor Laws* (1934), Appendix A.791 A.
40. *Extracts from the Information received by His Majesty's*

Commissioners as to the Administration and Operation of the Poor Laws (1833), pp. 115, 163, 216.

41. Hastings, p. 25.
42. *Royal Commission for Enquiry into the Administration and Practical Operation of the Poor Laws, 1834* (1905), pp. 51–4.
43. W. Scruton, *Pen & Pencil Pictures of Old Bradford* (Bradford, 1889), p. 113.
44. F. Healey, '40 Years of Resistance: The Reaction to the New Poor Law in the Todmorden Union 1834–1875', unpublished thesis, Halifax Local History Library, 1975, p. 64.
45. J. Wright, *The English Dialect Dictionary* (Oxford, 1961), vol. 1, p. 180.
46. F. W. Moorman, *Songs of the Ridings* (London, 1918), p. 24.
47. C. W. Hatfield, *Historical Notices of Doncaster* (Doncaster, 1866), pp. 313, 315.
48. Carlton Union Workhouse Papers, in Otley Museum.
49. *Leeds Board of Guardians Yearbook 1900–1901* (Leeds, 1900), pp. 24–5.
50. B. S. Rowntree, *Poverty, A Study in Town Life* (London, 1901), p. 98.
51. *Royal Commission on the Poor Laws and Relief of Distress* (1909), Appendix IV, pp. 266–7.
52. Moorman, pp. 34–5.
53. Notes in the Pontefract Museum Collection, generously made available by the Curator, Mr Richard Van Riel.

7.

Marching on their Stomachs:
The Soldier's Food in the
Nineteenth and Twentieth Centuries

H. G. MULLER

During the nineteenth and twentieth centuries there have been greater changes in the food supply of the British soldier than ever before in history. A number of well-documented incidents have been chosen because each was influenced by contemporary knowledge of food science, food technology, and nutrition.

The soldier's food has always been governed by four main factors. The first is the soldier's expectation. The British soldier's staple diet at the beginning of the nineteenth century was bread and boiled beef. By modern standards, his expectation was exceedingly low.

Modern Western troops have a very high expectation. The U.S. army tends to re-supply its troops with conventional food after three days of combat rations; Coca-Cola is often supplied free, perhaps as a marketing gesture. During the recent Gulf conflict some British journalists became separated from their troops. They were able to rejoin them by following a trail of empty tins of beans in tomato sauce and cartons of Jaffa Cakes.

Muslim soldiers expect *halal* meat, and some Hindus expect vegetarian fare. In Far Eastern wars involving, say, China or Korea, the soldiers may not expect anything more than a steady supply of rice. Food beyond that is a bonus. Guerrillas may expect no regular ration at all: they tend to live off the land.

The second factor is the level and consistency of provisioning. Even today it seems somewhat haphazard.

151

Compared with military hardware, food is relatively cheap and is often considered last. During a campaign supplies can be interrupted and this can result in difficulties. In Napoleon's day all transport was by horse and cart, as indeed it is today in many parts of the world. It is very slow, and the army can easily outrun it. In the Franco-German War of 1870–1, rail transport came into its own, but often huge bottlenecks arose at the railheads. The Second World War saw the rapid development of motor transport. Hitler built an excellent road network, but German motor transport was useless in the mud of Russia because there were insufficient tracked vehicles, and only these could move in the conditions.

The third factor to affect the soldier's food is the theatre of war. The climatic conditions, mainly temperature and relative humidity, can have pronounced effects on consumption and storage, particularly in the tropics. Sometimes, for example in desert warfare, water supply can become critical.

Finally, the state of food science, technology, and nutrition is of fundamental importance. The preservation of meat by drying and salting dates from ancient times, so too does the baking of bread and biscuits. Napoleon's soldiers, who are the earliest to be considered in this chapter, would have been quite familiar with these foods. Official rations were at a minimum, and the men had to depend on local purchase or plunder to satisfy their needs.

In the Crimean War dried vegetables became available, although the nutritional quality was poor. Being essentially a siege campaign, the soldiers in the Crimea were dependent upon official supply-lines, which tended to break down.

During the second part of the nineteenth century great advances in food processing were made. The work of Liebig and his school influenced nutrition, for example, in the Franco-German and the Boer Wars. The latter also saw the introduction of both canned and refrigerated meat for the troops.

In the First World War the research of U.S. and German scientists on energy metabolism was first applied. Operational Ration Packs (ORPs) were introduced in the Second World War, and the U.S. 'Meals Ready to Eat' (MREs) had their first serious test in the Gulf War, although that war was too short to evaluate them properly.

During the First Italian Campaign (1799) Napoleon's troops thoroughly plundered and pillaged northern Italy. Under the original plunder system the soldiers, individually or in small groups, would go out at the end of the day in search of food and fuel. By the sixteenth century, plunder became more organised. A party led by officers would move ahead, gather as much food and fuel as could be obtained, and then wait for the main body of men. As late as 1864, in the American Civil War, General Sherman's march through Georgia is a classic example. Each column sent out foragers into the rich and mainly agricultural state to pick up all food they could find.

The Napoleonic Wars

The plunder system, at least in India, was still accepted in 1914. The *Field Service Pocket Book* of that year[1] explains:

When foraging across the Indian frontier, look for foodstuffs as follows:
Waziristan – Buried beneath the floor of their huts,
Baluchistan – Hidden in karezes and nullahs,
Tirah – Behind false walls in houses,
Swat, Bajaur and Buner – In partitions and compartments built onto side walls of houses,
Burma – In granaries in the fields, usually no concealment.

The advantage of the 'plunder system' is that it requires a minimum of transport. However, the disadvantages are great: units become disorganised, the local people become hostile, and, in the event of a retreat, there is no food in the already denuded territory. This must have been very serious for Napoleon's troops in their retreat from Moscow, because the men's rations were too low.

The forces under Napoleon's command were very large indeed, and so were the associated logistical problems. In the campaign of 1805 he had 170,000 troops, swollen by 80,000 volunteers. Often the soldiers were quartered on the local inhabitants. The daily ration was 1½ lb of bread, ½ lb of meat, 1 oz. of rice, or 2 oz. of dried fruit. The firewood had to be supplied by their hosts.[2]

It is difficult to evaluate this daily ration in modern terms. For beef or pork the energy content varies from about 150 to 750 Kcal, depending on fat content. In this study a value of 300 Kcal has been used (Note: all energy values are given as Kcal/100g of edible matter.[3 4])

Bread is assumed to have been made from stoneground wholemeal wheat flour at 200 Kcal. (A contemporary definition of the usual stone-milled flour was: a substance the colour of sack cloth, consisting of equal parts of bran and millstone grit!) The ration (including rice or dried fruit) gives an energy value of approximately 2,000 Kcal. This is very low, and moreover is deficient in several micro-nutrients, particularly folate, lysine, and vitamins C and A. No doubt the soldier was expected to make up the shortfall.

At one stage in Napoleon's advance he ordered 500,000 biscuit rations to be prepared at Strasbourg and 200,000 at Mainz. Biscuits have been used on the continent of Europe for hundreds of years. Because of their low moisture content they can be kept for a long time and remain edible. A contemporary British military factory for biscuit manufacture was at Gosport. There were nine ovens and to each was attached a gang of five men. One, with his naked arms, mixed the dough from flour and water. The dough was then taken to a wooden platform called the break. It was there worked by a long pole, 7 ft long and fitted loosely to the wall at one end. The breakman worked this lever, the 'break staff', to and fro by jumping or sitting on the free end. When the dough had been kneaded in this way, it was shaped, stamped with a broad arrow and the number of the oven, and then baked. Since the baking time was short and seventy biscuits were baked at one time in the peel oven, the biscuits thrown in first had to be thicker than those inserted last. Only in the 1830s was the process mechanised with the introduction of mechanical mixers, 'breaker rollers' [*sic*], and docking machines. In this way production was increased from 1,500 to 2,240 lb of biscuits per hour. At the same time the operatives were reduced from forty-five to sixteen.[5]

King Charles I instituted Commissaries subject to Treasury control. These were stationed overseas where they represented the Treasury. They were responsible for the local purchase of supplies, placing contracts, paying bills and pensions, and controlling government transport. The sutlers, private entrepreneurs, supplied other requirements of food and drink, as they had done for centuries.[6][7]

During the Peninsular War (1808–14) Wellington made a careful study of supplies. He used to say that, besides being a General, he was a first-rate commissariat officer. Nevertheless, Wellington did not always find it easy to supply his troops. During and after the battle of Talavera (1809) provisions ran out. The daily ration consisted of ½ lb of wheat in the grain, and twice a week a few ounces of flour with ¼ oz. of goats' meat. The goats had first to be caught in the hills.

Mainly due to the war reporting of William Russell for the *London Times*, the public became aware during the Crimean War, perhaps for the first time, of the atrocious conditions under which the ordinary soldier had to operate. The commissariat was transferred from the Treasury to a 'Military Train', the forerunner of the Army Service Corps (ASC). Bakeries and butcheries were set up; and grocery supplies such as tea, coffee, pepper, and salt were bought in bulk. 'Bread-biscuits', baked as flat cakes and made of three

The Crimean War (1854–6)

155

14.
Crimea, 1854–6.
This cooking scene
must have been
familiar to soldiers
throughout many
centuries.

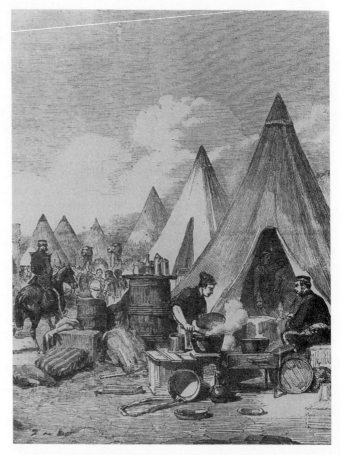

parts flour and one of peameal, arrived daily by boat from Constantinople. They soaked well in tea, coffee, or soup.

Alexis Soyer, a well-known chef and writer on culinary matters, visited the Crimea during the war. Meeting Miss Nightingale, 'the Lady with the Lamp', he immediately commented on the poor quality of the charcoal which 'smoked terribly and was nothing but dust'. The quality of the meat was also poor. It was either salted or obtained from cattle shipped in live. He soon improved the quality of the meals, and opened a large kitchen to his design at the Barrack Hospital, Miss Nightingale's hospital, in Skutary, on Easter Monday, 1855. Next, he modified the composition of the dried vegetable. Instead of just one, he suggested a spiced mixture of several: carrots, turnips, parsnips, and onions.

Cooking, both outside and inside tents, had been done on braziers or tripods from which kettles were suspended over the fire by a chain. Soyer designed a field stove (for which he became famous), which he later patented and which replaced cookery in the relatively small tin camp kettles. The cauldron could be removed and a false bottom placed over the fire to bake the bread. The stove could also be used for frying.

In his book, *Soyer's Culinary Campaign*,[8] Soyer gives twenty-one recipes of meals for between two and 1,000 men. Two examples follow:

No. One. *Soyer's Receipt to Cook Salt Meat for*
　　　　50 Men.
　　　　Put 50 lbs of meat in the boiler.
　　　　Fill with water and let soak overnight.
　　　　Next morning wash meat well.
　　　　Fill with fresh water, boil gently for three
　　　　hours and serve.

No. Six. *To Cook for a Regiment of 1,000 Men.*
　　　　Place 20 stoves in the open air or under
　　　　cover. Put 30 quarts of water in each
　　　　boiler, 50 lbs of ration meat, 4 squares of a
　　　　cake of dried vegetables – or if fresh mixed
　　　　vegetables are issued 12 lbs weight.
　　　　10 small tablespoons of salt, one ditto
　　　　pepper.
　　　　Light the fire and simmer gently for two to
　　　　two and a half hours. Skim the fat off the
　　　　top and serve.

15.
Alexis Soyer in
conversation with
two officers: his
field stoves are on
the right (Crimea,
(1854–6), from
A. Soyer, *Soyer's
Culinary Campaign*
(London, 1857).

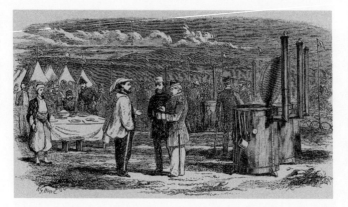

15.
Alexis Soyer in conversation with two officers: his field stoves are on the right (Crimea, (1854–6), from A. Soyer, *Soyer's Culinary Campaign* (London, 1857).

The process of preparing the compressed vegetable was based on the invention of the Frenchman Etienne Masson (Pat. No. 13338, 1850). The vegetable was dried in wicker trays in a current of warm air (75–145°F). Chemicals such as lime or calcium chloride were used to speed up the process. A partial vacuum could also be employed. The dried vegetable was then compressed, wrapped in tinfoil, and sealed into tins.

The field ration was as follows:[9]

		g	Kcal/100g	Kcal total
1½ lb	Bread	680	200	1,360
1 lb	Meat	454	300	1,360
2 oz.	Rice	57	350	200
2 oz.	Sugar	57	400	250
3 oz.	Coffee	85	300	250
1 gill	Spirits	140 ml	200	280
½ oz.	Salt	14	–	–

TOTAL 3,700

The energy level of this ration is satisfactory, but the lack of vitamin C, which causes scurvy, is striking.

The first cures for scurvy were purely empirical. In 1536 Jacques Cartier, the explorer, cured it among his sailors by an infusion of green leaves. In 1601 Captain James

Lancaster described lemon juice as a protective, and in 1747 James Lind actually cured the disease by the use of citrus fruit. In 1795 lemon juice was officially introduced into the British navy as a prophylactic. (For fuller details of the history of scurvy in the British navy, see Chapter 4.)

The stimulating effect of coffee had been recognised. However, coffee beans were supplied unroasted, which was characteristic of the general incompetence of those responsible for supply. The soldiers had no utensils for roasting, none for grinding, and were short of fuel. (Incidentally, coffee had been introduced into the American army ration already in 1832 to replace 4 oz. of spirit. Water-soluble instant coffee was introduced in the First World War and became very popular; it was mass-marketed in the Second World War. Freeze-dried coffee was first used in the Korean War.)

For the first nine months of the Crimean campaign there was no bread. This problem was eventually overcome by the construction of a floating mill and a floating bakery (Gaunt and Jones, *The Soldier's Food*).

Although certainly not the cause, the pretext for the mutiny was the issue of new paper cartridges. In order to charge a muzzle-loading musket, the soldier held the gun in his right hand, barrel upwards, and the paper cartridge in his left. He then tore off the twisted paper with his teeth and poured the gunpowder down the barrel. The cartridge, now containing only the bullet, was reversed and pushed down the barrel with the ramrod. After pulling back the hammer and applying the percussion cap to the nipple, the soldier had his musket ready to fire. (The very first health regulation for potential recruits was Napoleon's order that all men had to have sufficient teeth to tear their cartridges with ease.)

The Indian Mutiny (1857–9)

The problem with the new Enfield cartridge was the fact that it was coated with a mixture of beef and pork fat to make it reasonably moisture-proof. However, cows were sacred to Hindu soldiers, and pork is *haram* (forbidden) to

16.
The Enfield paper
cartridge: complete
(left), and cut open
to show the bullet
(right). Photograph
by H. G. Muller.

Muslims. Neither would place the cartridge in their mouths, and so the Indian Mutiny (or the First Indian War of Independence) began.

**The Franco-
German
Campaign
(1870–1)**

The American Civil War was the first modern conflict involving millions of men. The Franco-German campaign was the second. The task of feeding such an enormous body of men was accomplished largely by the use of the railways. Rail development had a very important impact on military transport. Food could easily be moved in large amounts, but flexibility decreased. In the American Civil War, the Confederate supply was dependent on just two railway lines. When these were captured, the supply system collapsed.

In the Franco-German Campaign, enormous jams arose on the German railway lines, which sometimes became blocked for hundreds of miles. Also the railheads, from which the food had to be collected by horse-drawn carts, often became a bottle-neck, and vast quantities of food were spoiled.

To appreciate the amounts of food required, one must remember the daily quantities involved (according to Gaunt and Jones, *The Soldier's Food*, p. 14):

148,000 3 lb loaves of bread;
102,000 lb of rice;
539 oxen, or 102,000 lb of bacon;
14,000 lb of salt;
28,000 quarts of spirits.

Additionally there were large amounts of coffee, sugar, and thousands of cigars. Every day, each army corps required five railway trains of thirty-two wagons each, to move all this food (Gaunt and Jones, *The Soldier's Food*).

The first half of the nineteenth century had seen a consolidation of nutritional science under the leadership of Justus von Liebig. In 1843 he wrote a popular book as a selection of letters 'for the special purpose of exciting the attention of governments'.[10] He divided all foods into plastic elements of nutrition (proteins) and elements of respiration (carbohydrates and fats). Among the former he listed: vegetable albumen, animal flesh, and animal blood. Among the elements of respiration he gave fat, starch, cane sugar, beer, and spirits.

The German soldier's daily ration[11] was:

	Kcal/100g	Kcal total
Meat 500g	300	1,500
Bread 750g	200	1,500
Bacon fat 250g	900	2,250
Beer 1l	50	500
Coffee 30g	300	90
Tobacco 60g	—	—
	Total	5,840

This ration reflects Liebig's work. There is a considerable increase in energy input, largely due to the addition of bacon fat.

Van Creveld (*Supplying War, Logistics from Wallenstein to Patton*) writes that the German troops often had to live off the rich agricultural countryside of France. Local supplies could be obtained as long as the army was on the march. Once they stopped to besiege (say, Paris or Metz), supply problems arose. Considering the soldiers' diet, it can safely be said that it was adequate as long as the army had access to additional local food. If they had to depend on army rations alone, the nutritional status of the men would have been seriously undermined, even if there had been no supply problems.

The Boer War (1899–1902)

Compared with the Crimean War, the Boer War saw several nutritional innovations. The first was the use of meat concentrate for emergency foods (iron rations).

Apparently the first to evaporate meat broth in the laboratory were two French chemists, Joseph Proust and Antoine Parmentier (recipes for making similar products at home had already appeared in cookery books under the titles 'Veal glue' or 'portable soup'). The product was preserved either as a paste or as slabs of glue-like material. Liebig became involved in the large-scale manufacture of meat extract in 1848. He realised the commercial potential of utilising the vast South American cattle herds for European use. (There was at the time no refrigerated transport.) In 1862 George Giebert, an engineer from Brazil, met Liebig in Munich. Liebig gave his name to the venture, and Giebert began production in Fray Bentos in Uruguay. First, the meat was ground and broken down. The fat was then separated and the remainder filtered, subjected to vacuum evaporation, and canned. The industry probably reached its zenith in the 1880s and then declined, due mainly to the competition of refrigerated meat.

The chocolate industry also profited from Liebig's work

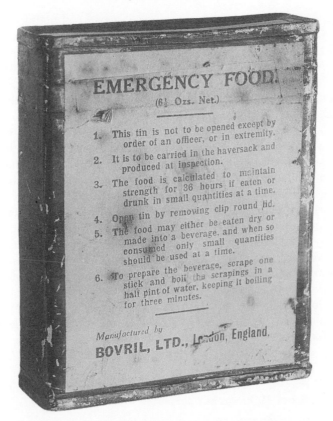

17.
Boer War iron
ration, *c.*1900.
Photograph by
courtesy of the
Science Museum,
London.

as it was well aware of chocolate's role in providing 'the
elements of respiration'. This is well illustrated in one of
the emergency ration packs of the Boer War. The canister
contained two tins: one held 4 oz. of beef concentrate; and
the other 5 oz. of cocoa paste.

The second innovation was the British soldiers' supply of
frozen meat. Frozen beef carcases can be transported with
greater ease and volume than live cattle, and large amounts
were supplied to the British forces in Southern Africa. It
was the US–Spanish War which saw the first use of
refrigerated transport. One of the first practical refrigeration

plants was designed by Henry and James Bell and J. J. Coleman. The Bell–Coleman patents were taken out in 1877, and the plants fitted to ships of the American, Australian, and later the New Zealand runs. In 1880 400 cwt. of frozen meat was imported into Britain from overseas. Only ten years later the amount imported annually had risen to 2.9 million cwt.

Finally, there was preserved meat in cans. Although it was the Frenchman Appert who studied the preservation in glass containers of various foods,[12] it was the London firm of Hall and Donkin who went into the mass production of cans of meat. A letter of Donkin dated 30 June 1817 survives in which he writes that he sold £3,000 of canned meat in the previous six months.

Since armies usually have to depend on ordinary trade commodities, only 6-lb cans were available because there was at that time little demand for smaller cans. The wooden boxes protecting the tin canisters were often used for firewood. There were also self-cooking rations, where the means of heating were contained in the same tin as the food. Large supplies of grain and cattle for slaughter were also obtained from Bechuanaland and Barotseland. At Mafeking the men received six weeks' full rations from local cattle and civilian stores. The dietary of the British soldier of 1900 was as follows:[13]

	Kcal/100g	Kcal total
454 g Meat	300	1,362
576 g Bread	200	1,152
227 g Fresh vegetables	10	23
85 g Sugar	400	340
19 g Coffee	300	57
14 g Salt	—	—
1 g Pepper	—	—
113 g Jam	250	283
71 ml Spirits	200	142
	Total	3,359

Compared with the daily ration of the Crimean War, the amount of meat was the same. Bread, coffee, and spirits had been reduced, but 'Liebig's elements of respiration' had been increased in the form of sugar and jam. Nutritionally noteworthy is the inclusion of fresh vegetables, although compressed vegetable was still available.

Masson's drying process of the Crimean War had been improved by Buchannan to a method whereby moisture was removed at reduced rather than elevated temperature. This would have tended to preserve vitamin C. Although the Board of Trade had recommended in 1871 that preserved rather than dried and compressed vegetables be used on board ship, according to Amery (*The Times History of the War in South Africa, 1899–1902*) such vegetables were still used by the army in the Boer War.

As always, the supply situation depended on the theatre of war, and whether the troops were on the move or in the trenches. In France, supplies were brought forward by train, and butcheries and bakeries were built at the railhead. The men of the Army Service Corps picked up bread and tins of corned beef by lorry, and took them to the men in the trenches, often under fire. Other supplies included canned jam, cheese, and prepared meals.

The First World War (1914–18)

There had been a large increase in meat canning, particularly in Australia and New Zealand, and much of it was produced as corned beef. To prepare this, the meat was finely divided and freed from sinews and fat. It was then salt-pickled and cooked. Next, it was forced into the cans by steam pressure and sealed. The cans were then left in boiling water for three to six hours, after which they were pierced to allow the water and fat to escape. Finally, the cans were again placed into boiling water for several hours.[14] In the German army, however, meat tended to be preserved as sausages rather than in cans.

In the event of active service, according to the *British*

18.
The 'Aldershot' oven was often used by the British Army, 1914–18. Photograph from author's collection.

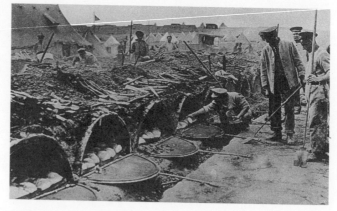

Field Service Pocket Book, the War Office gave the following daily ration as a guide:

	g	Kcal/100g	Kcal total
1¼ lb Meat	567	300	1,701
1¼ lb Bread	567	200	1,134
¼ lb Bacon	113	447	505
3 oz. Cheese	85	350	298
⅜ oz. Tea	18	100	18
¼ lb Jam	113	250	283
3 oz. Sugar	85	400	340
½ oz. Salt	14	—	—
1⁄36 oz. Pepper	1	—	—
1⁄20 oz. Mustard	1	—	—
½ lb Fresh veg.	227	10	23
½ gill Rum	71 ml	200	142
		Total	4,444

The energy content of bread is given as 200 Kcal, as before, assuming it to have been wholemeal. With the replacement of millstones by rollermills and the introduction of the 'gradual reduction process',[15] white bread would have been available. Its energy content would have been 233 Kcal because of the more efficient removal of bran. If fresh meat had been replaced by corned beef, the energy content would have been of the order of 217 Kcal because of the partial removal of fat.

The dietary stated further that if the 1½ lb of fresh vegetables had to be replaced by 2 oz. of dried vegetables, then ⅒ gill (14 ml) of lime juice had to be given. The destruction of vitamin C during the drying of the vegetables had therefore been clearly recognised and the vitamin added to compensate. (It was only late in 1916 that the superiority of lemon juice over lime juice as an anti-scorbutic was finally accepted, and the War Office amended its dietary instructions accordingly.) For simplicity, alternatives given in the dietary (e.g. salt meat for fresh, flour for bread) have been omitted.

For Aden camel drivers the following dietary was suggested:

	g	Kcal/100g	Kcal total
1½ lb Rice	680	350	2,380
1 lb Dates, wet	454	144	654
2 oz. Ghee	57	898	512
2 oz. Sugar	57	400	250
⅓ oz. Coffee	10	300	30
½ oz. Salt	14	—	—
4 oz. Dahl	113	347	392
		Total	4,218

The South African native's ration was to be:

	g	Kcal/100g	Kcal total
1½ lb Maize meal	680	360	2,448
1½ lb Meat	680	300	2,040
½ oz. Salt	14	—	—
		Total	4,488

Although these three dietaries are completely different, the energy content is remarkably similar.

Energy studies on foods had begun already with Lavoisier in the 1790s, and continued with Deprez and Dulon in the

19.
Mobile German
army bakeries of
the First World
War, 1914–18.
Photograph from
author's collection.

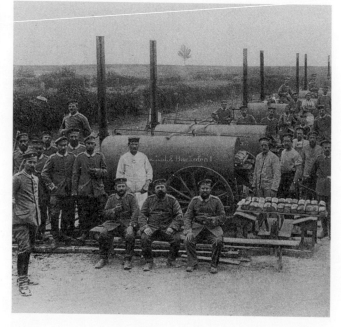

1820s. These researches led to the work of Pettenkover and Voit, who designed a calorimeter for studies of basal metabolism in 1861. In 1904 Atwater and Benedict used their respiration calorimeter in studies of human nutrition. Such studies were further advanced after 1907, when F. G. Benedict began thirty years of research on energy metabolism and respiration calorimetry at the nutrition laboratory of the Carnegie Institute at Boston.[16] It is apparent that some of this work was already being utilised in the preparation of the three dietaries.

The *British Field Service Pocket Book* of 1914 also gives eighteen recipes. The simplest are for chapaties and kebabs. Those for soups and stews are more complicated and time-consuming. The only sweet is plain rice pudding.

During the war the need for a nutritional analysis of the

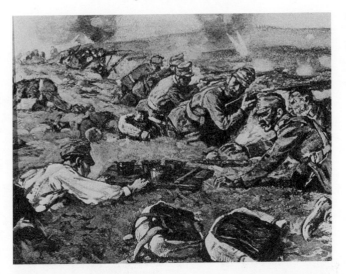

20.
Austrian soldiers
receiving their meal
under fire, 1914.
Photograph from
author's collection.

more common foods eaten in Britain became urgent, because
the army, as well as the rest of the community, was strictly
rationed. The task was given to Capt R. H. A. Plimmer, a
recognised authority on analytical technique. Apart from
being attached to the War Office, he was also head of the
Biochemistry department at the Rowett Research Institute
of the University of Aberdeen. He later became Professor of
Chemistry at University College, London, and together with
his wife Violet published a very popular small book on
vitamins, which in his day were the main topic of food
research.[17] He prepared a report of about 250 pages of
tables for the use of the Army Medical Authorities,
published by Her Majesty's Stationery Office in 1921. In
the appendix he gave a semi-quantitative assessment of the
three vitamins known at the time: A, B, and C.[18]

During and before the First World War the British soldier **The Second**
obtained two reasonable meals and one meagre meal a day. **World War**
Cooks were largely untrained, and could spoil the food even **(1939–45)**

21.
A kitchen scene in
the First World
War. The soldier on
the left is chopping
wood. In the
background the men
are cutting up meat.
The man on the
right slices bread.
Behind the flagon in
the centre is a dish
with eggs, and in
front some tins,
probably of jam.
Photograph from
author's collection.

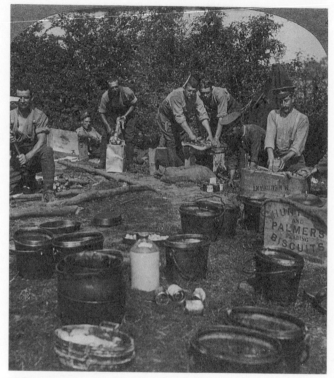

if the original raw materials were satisfactory. A reform in
1930 increased the meal allowance, and the soldiers were
able to obtain four meals, which were also of better quality,
every day.

In 1938 Sir Isidore Salmon, Chairman and Managing
Director of J. Lyons, caterers well known for the Lyons
Corner House, became the honorary catering adviser to the
army. He suggested improved methods of catering and
better training methods for the cooks, and these were quickly
adopted. However, a real revolution in army catering
occurred in 1941 with the creation of the Army Catering

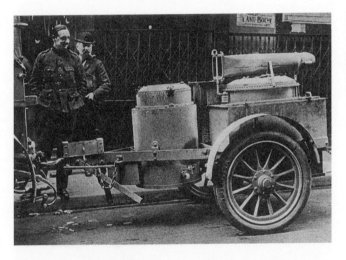

22.
A Belgian field kitchen of 1916, the descendant of Soyer's field stove. Photograph from author's collection.

Corps. All army cooks were transferred to it. It also became responsible for their training and for general administration.

The first quarter of the twentieth century had seen great activity in the search for accessory food factors. By 1913 a fat-soluble, and by 1915 a water-soluble essential food factor had been discovered. In 1916 these were named 'fat-soluble A' and 'water-soluble B' factors. Between 1919 and 1922 it became clear that the B factor consisted of more than one active component. By 1939 most of the important vitamins had been found (such as A, D, E, most of the B vitamins, and C).

Of the essential mineral elements, iron and calcium had long been known. Evidence of the essential role of other trace elements was found as follows: iodine, 1895; phosphorus, 1918; copper, 1928; magnesium and manganese, 1931; zinc, 1933; and cobalt, 1935. With the recognition of this large number of accessory food factors, the range of food for the military was greatly increased.

The standard British service ration now consisted of 12 oz. of bread or 9 oz. of biscuits, 10 oz. of fresh meat, and no less than forty-two alternative foods such as fruit, vegetables, bacon, cheese, jam, and chocolate. Standard drinks were tea, coffee, and cocoa. Fresh produce was also purchased locally.[19] Special meals were provided for Jewish, Muslim, and Hindu soldiers.

The meals were often prepared behind the lines and, if hot, were taken to the front lines in insulated containers. One type of these was the 'hay box', where hay provided the insulation.[20][21]

The Second World War was the first war in which Operational Ration Packs (ORPs) were produced for the British army. The simplest of these was the Emergency Ration (Standard), which consisted of 6 oz. of a solid chocolate mixture in a small tin box. It was phased out in 1944 following the introduction of the various special ORPs.

Next came the Mess Tin Ration (48 hours). There were two water- and gas-proof packs which fitted into the mess tin. One contained biscuits, raisins, chocolate, and boiled sweets (24 ½ oz.); the other dripping spread, cheese, a tea/sugar/milk mixture, and preserved meat (22 oz.). Matches and a cooker were also supplied. There were 250,000 of these packs produced as airborne and seaborne landing rations to supply the soldier for the first 48 hours. However, since the pack proved to be too heavy in relation to nutritional value, the 24-hour ration pack was designed. Weight was reduced by replacing metal containers with waxed cardboard boxes. This pack contained biscuits, oatmeal, tea/sugar/milk blocks, a meat block, raisin chocolate, vitaminised chocolate, boiled sweets, chewing gum, cubes of meat extract, salt, sugar, and lavatory paper. It weighed 2 lb 3 oz. and had a nutritional value of approximately 4,000 Kcal.

The Composite 14-Men Pack (Compo) was designed for feeding troops for periods not exceeding six weeks, and it was to follow the consumption of the 24-hour pack. There were seven types (A to G) with biscuits, and three types (1, 2, and 3) to be issued when bread was available. There were

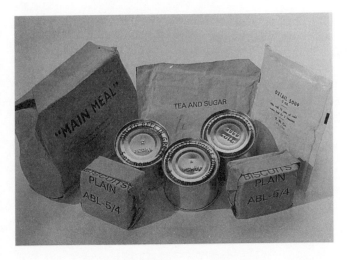

23.
Composite ration,
c.1970. Photograph
by H. G. Muller.

twenty items of food, as well as soap, matches, and lavatory paper. The energy value of A–G was about 3,590 Kcal and the gross weight 66 lb. Types 1–3 had an energy value of 3,520 Kcal, if taken with 14 oz. of bread per day.

Apart from these, there were special packs for Armoured Fighting Vehicles (AVFs). Here the weight was not of such importance. Airborne packs were designed for use by aircraft crews, and other packs had to fit into bomb-type containers for air drops. The energy content of all these packs was about 3,500 Kcal, except for the Mountain (Arctic) pack which contained 5,100 Kcal.

The American invasion of Europe was supported by three types of such pre-packed rations. The emergency D-ration consisted of a high-energy chocolate bar of 1,000 Kcal, made by Hershey, a well-known American chocolate manufacturer. The K-ration consisted of a tin of meat and a powdered synthetic drink, 'not popular in a muddy foxhole in freezing weather'.[22] It also contained crackers, cigarettes, lavatory paper, and later a fruit bar. Like the K-ration, the C-ration was lightweight. It contained small tins of

173

individual servings of soup or stew. B-rations were bulky and much larger than the individual packs.[23]

Plunder or barter was not unknown when food ran out, or official rations palled. Cows were shot, fish stunned with hand grenades, and poultry 'liberated'. A chocolate bar was exchanged for a bottle of wine and a Luger pistol was worth 10 lb of coffee.

The American steel helmet was well designed. The lining was fitted to a lightweight plastic helmet onto which the steel helmet could be placed. This latter, devoid of lining, could serve as a wash basin or cooking pot. Half a dozen eggs cooked in a GI helmet would be a rare treat.[24] The American GI's reaction to standard army fare was not always enthusiastic:

> The biscuits in the army
> they say are mighty fine.
> One fell off the table
> and killed a pal of mine.
>
> Oh, I've got enough of army life,
> gee, Mom, I want to go,
> but they won't let me go,
> gee, Mom, I want to go home.
>
> The coffee in the army
> they say is mighty fine.
> It tastes like disinfectant
> and smells of iodine.
>
> Anon.

The German army went into the war with a great deal of crisp bread, and dried vegetables ranging from potatoes and carrots to cabbage and sauerkraut. The vegetable was compressed into blocks, and wrapped in aluminium foil or cellophane. Yeast extract provided some B group vitamins, and tomato puree vitamin C. Short of tins, the Germans seem to have specialised in dried vegetables, also prepared for export. For instance, thousands of cases of dried potatoes were sent to British India, 40,000 kg to the British troops in the Boer War, and several wagon loads to France as late as March 1914.[25]

'Normal' and 'Special' rations were available, and in 1943 the Nutrition Laboratories of the Waffen-SS developed a 'Concentrate'. This was designed to combine the highest nutritive value with the lowest weight.[26] Heavy packaging (cans, tubes) was avoided. The 'Concentrate' consisted of three varieties:

a) sweet compounds: three types with about 25 per cent sucrose;
b) salty compounds: four types, two based on legumes, one each on rice and potatoes; and
c) beverages: coffee, tea.

In an appendix to E. G. Schenk, *Zur Frage der Sonder-und Konzentrat-Verpflegung der Waffen-SS, c.*1943, the US rations were evaluated. It was concluded that the raw material was excellent, but there was nothing new except a very good caramel-malt-skim milk sweet in some of the D rations, described as: 'Only slightly sweet, not sticky and dissolves only slowly in the mouth'. Finally, and as a portent of things to come, appeared the remark: 'Interesting, but not to be imitated, is the copious use of chemical preservatives and colour'.

The modern German army specifications (1985) are as follows:[27]

Group	Animal Protein g	Fat g	Energy Kcal	Vit. A mg	Vit. B mg	Vit. C mg
1	60	150	4,000	0.9	2.4	75
2	60	128	3,400	0.9	2.0	75
3	60	105	2,800	0.9	1.7	75
4	40	90	2,600	0.9	1.6	75

The group refers to:
1 Front-line troops, air force, and navy on active service
2 Reserve
3 Other army personnel
4 Non-working prisoners of war.

Some of the iron rations of various armies are given in a German publication of 1939 on soldiers' dietary and the provisioning of armies (see Table 1).

The Gulf Conflict (1991) The specifications of the Ministry of Defence (MoD) are strict (*Operational Ration Packs, Emergency Flying Rations, Survival Rations*, 1990). At present there are five Operational Ration Packs (ORPs), which were used in the Gulf Conflict by the British and which conform to the following:

Type	Number of menus	Protein	Fat	CHO	Kcal
			Energy derived from: (man/day)%		
10-man	7	12	36.0	52	3,480
4-man	7	12	36.0	52	3,880
24-hour GS	4	12	26.0	62	4,750
24-hour Arctic	4	12	26.0	62	4,750
24-hour GP	7	12	33.0	55	4,600

(Note: GS = general service for use mainly by patrols; GP = general purpose; CHO = carbohydrate. With the first two types biscuits or bread are given to provide the stated energy value. The 24-hour Arctic type was used in the Falklands War.)

It is apparent from this data that there are four or seven different menus for each type of ORP. Each daily menu consists of breakfast, a main meal, and tea. To give just one example: for the ten-man ORP, the breakfast list for the week (seven days) consists of sausages, bacon grill, baconburgers, baked beans in tomato sauce, and oatmeal blocks. All these are rotated, except for the baked beans, which are given every day.

On the 'main meal' list are twenty-three items, all of which are rotated daily. The meal on day one consists of: mushroom soup, goulash, carrots, mashed potato powder, and apple pudding; day two: mulligatawny soup, corned beef, mixed vegetables, again potato powder, and canned pears; day three: chicken soup, casserole steak and onions,

Table 1. Iron rations of ten national armies, 1939

	Holland g	USA g	Belgium g	France g	England g	Italy g	Romania g	Hungary g	Czechoslovakia g	Japan g
Beans	–	–	–	50	–	400	–	–	–	150 Miso
Canned meat	200	196	300	300	340	150	300	300	200	90 (smoked meat)
Canned mix	200	127	–	–	–	–	–	–	–	–
Smoked sausage	200	–	–	–	–	–	–	–	–	–
Cheese	500	185	500	–	–	–	–	200	200	–
Rusk or canned bread	750	–	–	450	454	400	500	200	–	690
Sugar	–	67	60	80	57	–	–	–	–	–
Coffee	–	17	45	36	–	–	10	54	80	–
Salt	–	–	20	–	–	–	4	20	–	–
Chocolate	–	84	–	125	–	–	–	–	–	–
Spirits	–	–	–	62	–	–	–	15	–	–
Tobacco	–	–	–	20	–	–	1	–	–	–
Tea	–	–	–	–	177	–	–	–	–	–
Rice	–	–	–	–	–	–	–	–	–	870 or 120 g rice bran

Source: W. Kittel, W. Schreiber and W. Ziegelmayer, *Soldatenernährung und Gemeinschaftsverpflegung* (Dresden 1939).

processed peas, potato powder, and mixed fruit pudding. day four: oxtail soup, chicken curry, carrots, milled rice, and fruit salad; day five: vegetable soup, steak and kidney pudding, processed peas, potatoes, and apple pudding; day six: oxtail soup, chicken in brown sauce, peas, rice and peaches; and day seven: vegetable soup, stewed steak, carrots, potatoes, and mixed fruit pudding. The meals are then repeated. Tea consists in rotation of one of the following main portions: luncheon meat, beefburgers, pilchards in tomato sauce, or rich cake. If heating is required, hexamine cookers are available.

The packs may be conventional cans of different sizes, Alucans, retortable pouches, or sachets. Alucans are semi-rigid aluminium containers which, unlike conventional cans, are heat-sealed and not seamed. Both types are processed in over-pressure retorts at 121°C. Time and pressure depend on the product. The process is tolerant of limited liquid contamination in the seal area.

Retortable pouches have certain advantages over conventional cans. They are lighter in weight and, being flat, they are easier to retort and so give a better quality product. They are usually 3-ply, with an outer layer of polyester, an aluminium layer in the middle, and an inner layer of polythene near the food to prevent any reaction with the content. In practice the seal is difficult because food or grease can enter it and there may be a problem with pinholes in the pouch itself. Nonetheless, some years ago, the US army awarded a contract for $21.3 million to the American Pouch Co. in order to develop pouches to replace the C-ration. Since then, retortable pouches have been greatly improved.

The shelf life of ORPs is usually about two to three years and therefore they are continually rotated. Quality control is conducted in special control laboratories in each major area where British forces serve. Purchase by the MoD is by tender. Wherever possible, standard packs or products manufactured by national food processors are used. Non-

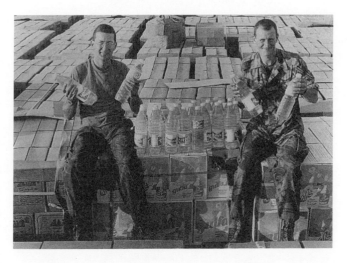

24.
Drinking water for the 'Squaddies', Gulf War, 1991. Photograph by courtesy of *Soldier* magazine.

standard products are disproportionately expensive.

During the Gulf War the US forces had twelve 'Meals Ready to Eat' (MREs), as well as crackers and packaged bread. One MRE consists of a single meal in a pouch for one man, together with plastic eating utensils and a moist towelette (see Baird, *Hot Meals in a Hot Spot*). French units had to cut their available choice of meals from fifteen to five, because in Muslim Saudi Arabia pork is not allowed. British and US forces still used pork because meals containing it were sealed in containers. It was also pointed out that: 'Desert Shield troops should not worry about the effect of MREs on sex drive or on the digestive system. . . . No chemicals are added to lessen libido and the meals do not cause constipation.'

I wish to thank Mr C. J. F. Townson of Evotec Limited and Lt. Col. G. Wilkinson for their kind advice.

Acknowledge-ment

Notes and References

1. *British Field Service Pocket Book* (London, 1914).
2. M. van Crefeld, *Supplying War. Logistics from Wallenstein to Patton* (Cambridge, 1990).

3. A. A. Paul and D. A. T. Southgate, *The Composition of Foods* (London, 1978).
4. S. P. Tan, R. W. Wenlock, and D. H. Buss, *Immigrant Foods* (London, 1985).
5. C. Tomlinson, *Cyclopaedia of Useful Arts* (London, 1853).
6. J. Fortescue, *Canteens in the British Army* (Cambridge, 1928).
7. J. Fortescue, *The Early History of Transport and Supply* (London, 1928).
8. A. Soyer, *Soyer's Culinary Campaign* (London, 1857).
9. F. A. Gaunt and C. J. A. Jones, *The Soldier's Food* ([Aldershot] Graphics Dept. STW HQ ACC TC, 1978).
10. J. von Liebig, *Familiar Letters on Chemistry* (London, 1843).
11. R. Russell, *Strength and Diet* (London, 1905).
12. N. Appert, *The Art of Preserving all Kinds of Animal and Vegetable Substances for Several Years* (London, 1811).
13. L. S. Amery, *The Times History of the War in South Africa 1899–1902*, vol. 6 (London, 1909), p. 382.
14. C. Ainsworth Mitchel, *Flesh Foods* (London, 1900).
15. W. R. Voller, *Modern Flour Milling* (Gloucester, 1889).
16. M. Swartz Rose, *The Foundations of Nutrition* (New York, 1933).
17. R. H. A. Plimmer and V. G. Plimmer, *Food, Health, Vitamins* (London, 1925).
18. R. H. A. Plimmer, *Analyses and Energy Values of Foods* (London, 1921).
19. I. S. O. Playfair, *The Mediterranean and the Middle East* vol. 6, pt 1 (London, 1984), pp. 450–4.
20. Anon., *Food Facts for the Kitchen Front* (London, 1941).
21. War Office, *Manual of Military Cooking and Dietary* pt 1, General (London, 1940).
22. W. Maulding, *Up Front* (Cleveland, 1946).
23. MoD, *UK Armed Services. Operational Ration Packs, Emergency Flying Rations, Survival Rations* (Bath, 1990).
24. B. Baird, 'Hot Meals in a Hot Spot', *Food Technology*, 45, pt 2 (1991), pp. 52–6.
25. W. Kittel, W. Schreiber, and W. Ziegelmayer, *Soldatenernährung und Gemeinschaftsverpflegung* (Dresden, 1939).
26. E. G. Schenk, *Zur Frage der Sonder- und Konzentrat-Verpflegung der Waffen-SS* (SS-Wirtschafts-Verwaltungshauptamt, Amtsgruppe B, undated, c.1943).
27. Bundesamt für Wehrtechnik und Beschaffung, *Verteidigungsvorrat, Verpflegung und Feldverpflegungsgerät der Bundeswehr* (Bundesamt für Wehrtechnik und Beschaffung, 5400 Koblenz, 1985).

Index

181

Index

Index

Index

vegetables, 59, 89-90, 108-9
  monastic diet, 10, 13, 17, 25
  soldiers, 152, 157, 158, 165, 167
Vernon, Admiral, 85
viande, 101
vinegar, 72, 84
vitamins
  A, 169
  B, 91, 169
  C, 10, 71, 84, 90-1, 158, 165-9

wafers, 18
wages, 48-9, 51-2, 54-7, 91 n.1
walnuts, pickled, 94 n.42
Waltham Abbey, 18
water, 75, 79, 84, 99-101, 110, 152
Waverley Abbey, 15, 33
weevils, 83, 87, 93 n.29
welfare state, 146
Wellington, Duke of, 155
West Riding, Yorkshire, 126, 137
wheat, 18, 22-3, 50, 53, 106
Whitsuntide, 129
Wickwane, Archbishop, 14
wine
  monastic diet, 9, 12, 13, 27
  sailors, 79, 85
  Saint Cyr, 106, 110, 114
  servants, 46, 48, 49

women
  Monasteries, 40-1 n.49
  servants, 44, 50-2, 55, 58, 62
  workhouses, 135, 141, 145
Woodforde, Parson, 65
workhouses, 3, 116-50
  Beverley, 122-3, 124
  Bradford, 137, 145
  Carlton, 138-9
  Doncaster, 125, 138
  Ecclesfield, 127, 128
  Halifax, 122, 128
  Headingley, 128
  Hedon, 134-5
  Horbury, 125
  Hull, 122, 127, 128
  Kidderminster, 136
  Knaresborough, 129
  Leeds, 123-5, 127-30, 135, 143-4
  Ovenden, 127, 128, 131-3
  Oxford, 135-6
  Pocklington, 127
  Pontefract, 139-40, 148
  Pudsey, 131
  Scarborough, 136
  Sheffield, 127, 128, 129, 130-1
  Southowram, 128
  Todmorden, 137
  Wharfedale, 138-9, 141-2

York, 117, 119, 120, 126
Yorke family, 56, 58, 63, 64
Young, Reverend George, 133-4

185